Study Guide
to Accompany

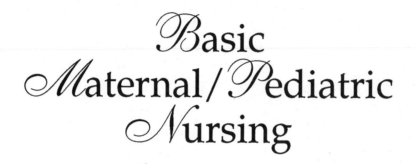

Basic
Maternal/Pediatric
Nursing

Pamela J. Shapiro, BSN, ARNP
Ann Sinisi Scott, RN, MS

NOTICE TO THE READER

COPYRIGHT © 1995
By Delmar Publishers
an International Thomson Publishing Company

The ITP logo is a trademark under license.

Printed in the United States of America

For more information contact:

Delmar Publishers
3 Columbia Circle, Box 15015
Albany, New York 12212-5015

International Thomson Publishing
Berkshire House
168-173 High Holborn
London, WC1V7AA
England

International Thomson Publishing Gmbh
Konigswinterer Str. 418
53227 Bonn
Germany

Thomson Nelson Australia
102 Dodds Street
South Melbourne 3205
Victoria, Australia

International Thomson Publishing Asia
221 Henderson Bldg. #05-10
Singapore 0315

International Thomson Publishing Japan
Kyowa Building, 3F
2-2-1 Kirakawa-cho
Chiyoda-ku, Tokyo 102
Japan

Nelson Canada
1120 Birchmont Road
Scarborough, Ontario
M1K 5G4, Canada

1 2 3 4 5 6 7 8 9 10 XXX 01 00 99 98 97 96 95 94

ISBN: 0-8273-6354-0
Library of Congress Catalog Card Number: 94-19097

To the Student

This study guide has been prepared for students using the text *Basic Maternal/Pediatric Nursing*. With this study guide, students can review concepts and information presented in the textbook and also theoretically apply these concepts through activities, exercises, and case studies.

Page references to the text are printed in the left margin next to each question. These text references allow you to review or confirm answers.

The pages of this study guide are three-hole punched and perforated to allow easy removal of pages if your instructor wishes to collect completed assignments for evaluation purposes. You may want to use a three-ring notebook to store completed assignments for easy reference and review. The answers to the questions are included in your teacher's Instructor's Guide. See your teacher if you have difficulty with any of the questions in this study guide.

The authors hope you find this study guide to be both challenging and interesting. It is our desire that you master the content of the text to the best of your ability, and we believe this study guide will assist you in that process.

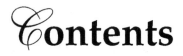ontents

CHAPTER

1

The History of Maternal/Newborn Nursing

MULTIPLE CHOICE
Select the one best answer.

4 1. The first U.S. ordinance dealing with the ethical conduct of midwives occurred in

    a. 1621   c. 1716
    b. 1660   d. 1910

4 2. What percentage of births was reported by midwives in 1910?

    a. 25%   c. 50%
    b. 33%   d. 62%

6 3. AWHONN is an organization that provides all of the following services except:

    a. certification of women's health nurse practitioners
    b. a bimonthly professional journal
    c. educational programs
    d. health insurance programs

7 4. The consumer has influenced the labor and delivery experience in all of the following ways except

    a. requesting more information about medical procedures
    b. requesting partners be in attendance during labor and delivery
    c. requesting a more homelike atmosphere in the hospital setting
    d. requesting more frequent use of nurse midwives

1

3   5. Nutricius is a Latin term meaning all of the following except
        a.   to conserve energy
        b.   to protect
        c.   to nourish
        d.   to nurse

3   6. The chief purpose of nursing today is to
        a.   carry out the physician's orders
        b.   help people attain or maintain health
        c.   dispense medication and assist in procedures that promote wellness
        d.   specialize in a distinct field of medicine

6   7. All of the following about the nurse practitioner in women's health care are true
        except that they
        a.   have advanced education
        b.   have been certified by a special board
        c.   carry out many of the functions of a physician
        d.   must always be supervised by a physician

3   8. The nurse who was influential in organizing the American Red Cross was
        a.   Bridget Lee Fuller
        b.   Florence Nightingale
        c.   Clara Barton
        d.   Anne Hutchinson

6   9. There was a dramatic decrease in maternal and infant mortality after 1935 due to
        a.   better midwifery training
        b.   better physician training
        c.   an increased trend toward hospital births
        d.   the use of medication

5   10. The construction of hospitals in rural areas to accommodate women who did not
        have access to a hospital to give birth was accomplished by the
        a.   Brown-Hill Act
        b.   Hill-Burton Act
        c.   Aldridge Construction Bill
        d.   Anne Hutchinson Act

SHORT ANSWER

3–4   1. List three prominent midwives in history.

     a. _Fuller_

     b. _Hutchinson_

     c. _____

7   2. Name three individuals influential in training expectant mothers to be prepared for the labor and delivery process.

     a. _Lamaze_

     b. _Dick-Read_

     c. _Bradley_

7–9   3. List four differences found in an alternative birthing center (ABC) that would not be found in the traditional hospital facility.

     a. _Birthing Rooms_

     b. _____

     c. _____

     d. _____

7   4. State the purpose of prepared childbirth classes.

3   5. List five qualities a nurse should possess.

     a. _Knowledge_

     b. _Ability to understand & adjust_

     c. _Social & behavioral science_

     d. _teacher_

     e. _attain & maintain health_

MATCHING

Match the terms in the left column with their definitions in the right column.

4	_____	a.	Maternity Center Association in New York City began teaching midwives
3	_____	b.	midwifery book published by Rodienm
4	_____	c.	first occurrence of midwifery in the United States
4	_____	d.	Anne Hutchinson massacred by the Indians
3	_____	e.	first formal training for midwives
4	_____	f.	legal regulation of midwifery standards began
3	_____	g.	Loyse Boursier was midwife to the French Court
4	_____	h.	Anne Hutchinson was condemned for interpretation of the Bible
4	_____	i.	New York state midwifery law transferred control of midwives to city's board of health
4	_____	j.	50% of all births were delivered by midwives
6	_____	k.	certification of nurse practitioners

1. fifth century B.C.
2. 1513
3. 1563–1636
4. 1621
5. 1637
6. 1643
7. 1716
8. 1907
9. 1910
10. 1915
11. 1976

EXERCISES

1. Select a nurse or midwife in history, and write a brief report about her life and accomplishments.

2. Research and write a brief report about how maternity care has changed, starting with the early midwifery and home birth period, and include the present ABC and birthing room concepts.

CHAPTER

2

The Female Reproductive System

MULTIPLE CHOICE
Select the one best answer.

15–16   1. Which of the following is *not* a part of the vulva?
    a. labia majora and labia minora
    b. clitoris
    c. vagina
    d. Bartholin gland

15–16   2. Which of the following statements about the clitoris is not correct?
    a. The clitoris is homologous to the male scrotum.
    b. The clitoris is an elongated mass of tissue, nerves, and muscle.
    c. The clitoris is homologous with the male penis.
    d. The clitoris is extremely sensitive to sexual excitement.

16   3. The anterior and posterior boundaries of the perineum are the
    a. vulva and the anus
    b. mons pubis and the vaginal opening
    c. vaginal opening and the anus
    d. urethra and the anus

16   4. Which of the following statements about the vagina is incorrect?
    a. It is internally situated between the bladder and the rectum.
    b. It is an excretory duct for the uterus.
    c. It is lined with folds called rugae.
    d. It is rich in nerve endings and very sensitive to sexual stimulation.

5. The normal place for conception to occur is
   a. in the uterus
   b. in the outer one-third of the fallopian tube
   c. in the inner quarter of the fallopian tube
   d. on the surface of the ovary after the ovum has matured

6. The female sex gland(s) is/are the
   a. uterus   c. ovaries
   b. clitoris   d. pituitary

7. The process by which a mature ovum is released and made ready to receive the fertilized ovum is called
   a. menstruation   c. ovulation
   b. procreation   d. fertilization

8. Gonadotropin-releasing hormone is produced by the
   a. pituitary   c. ovary
   b. hypothalamus   d. uterus

9. Follicle-stimulating hormone is produced by the
   a. pituitary   c. ovary
   b. hypothalamus   d. uterus

10. The luteinizing hormone is produced by the
    a. pituitary   c. ovary
    b. hypothalamus   d. uterus

11. Estrogen is produced by the
    a. pituitary   c. ovary
    b. hypothalamus   d. uterus

12. Progesterone is produced by the
    a. pituitary   c. ovary
    b. hypothalamus   d. uterus

13. The false pelvis is composed of the
    a. lower part of the pelvis   c. upper flaring part of the pelvis
    b. pelvic brim   d. pubis and ischium

14. Milk-producing cells in the breast tissue are called
    a. acini   c. ducts
    b. lobes   d. alveoli

20   15. Menstrual flow consists of all of the following except

      a. blood   c. mucous secretions

      b. tissue fragments   (d.) cilia

SHORT ANSWER

15   1. List four functions of the female reproductive system.

      a. *produce hormones*

      b. *" ovum + environment for conception*

      c. *nurture & sustain develop. fertilized ovum*

      d. *to accomplish delivery of product of conception*

16   2. Name the three sections that make up the uterus.

      a. *fundus*

      b. *body* } *uterus*

      c. *cervix*

17   3. Name three distinct parts of the cervix.

      a. *cervix canal*

      b. *internal os*

      c. *external os*

18–19   4. What three structures do the broad ligaments support? *pelvic organs*

      a. _____

      b. _____ *p 19*

      c. _____

20   5. Describe the follicular/proliferative phase of the menstrual cycle.

20   6. Describe the luteal/secretory phase of the menstrual cycle.

23   7. Name the three innominate bones that form the pelvis.
       a. _ilium_
       b. _pubis_
       c. _ischum_

20   8. Name two functions of the ovaries.
       a. _to mature & discharge ova_
       b. _To produce hormones to process of reproduction_

25   9. Define puberty.
       12-18 Of to reproduce

25   10. Define menopause.
       permanent cessation
       of menstrual flow

MATCHING

1. Match the following terms with their definitions.

22   _3_   a. amenorrhea   1. painful menstruation
23   _5_   b. menorrhagia   2. bleeding at irregular times
23   _2_   c. metrorrhagia   3. absence of menses
23   _1_   d. dysmenorrhea   4. menstruation without ovulation
23   _4_   e. anovulation   5. excessive bleeding

2. Match the following pelvic shapes with their descriptions.

23–24

_3_   a. gynecoid ✗   1. heart or wedge shape

_1_   b. android   2. flattened pelvis

_4_   c. anthropoid ✗   3. round or transverse oval

_2_   d. platypelloid   4. narrow transverse plane with greater anteroposterior diameter

LABELING

Label the following female external anatomical structures.

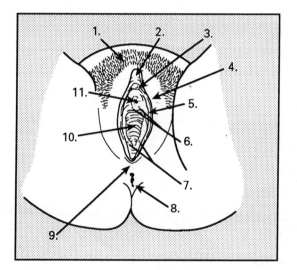

1. _Mons pubis_   7. _Bartholin's Ducts_

2. _Prepuce_   8. _Anus_

3. _Clitoris_   9. _perineum_

4. _Labia majora_   10. _Vagina_

5. _Labia minora_   11. _meatus_

6. _Skene's Ducts_

CASE STUDIES

1. Mary is a 22-year-old woman who comes to the clinic for her yearly examination and Pap smear. She and her husband are considering a pregnancy in the near future, but Mary states she knows little about the best time to attempt conception. She asks the nurse to educate her about fertility awareness.

   a. What information is necessary for the nurse to obtain from Mary before she can answer her question?

   b. Assuming Mary has regular menses, how should the nurse explain fertility awareness to Mary?

2. Elizabeth is a 52-year-old woman who presents with complaints of severe mood swings, hot flashes, night sweats, and vaginal dryness. She is frightened by these changes in her system and thinks she may have a threatening disease.

   a. What additional information should the nurse obtain from Elizabeth?

   b. What is the probable cause of Elizabeth's symptoms?

   c. What can the nurse tell Elizabeth to alleviate her fears?

CHAPTER

3

Conception

MULTIPLE CHOICE
Select the one best answer.

32   1. The external sex organs of the male are the
      a. penis and the scrotum
      b. testicles and the penis
      c. glans penis and the dartos
      d. epididymis and the testis

32–33   2. Semen is a mixture of secretions from all of the following structures except the
      a. testes and prostate
      b. seminal vesicles and testes
      c. bulbourethral glands and seminal vesicles
      d. cavernous bodies and urethra

33   3. The principal storehouse for sperm is/are the
      a. testes   c. seminiferous tubules
      b. epididymis   d. vas deferens

33   4. Male gonadotropic hormones are released from the
      a. hypothalamus   c. testes
      b. pituitary   d. Cowper's glands

33   5. Testosterone contributes to all of the following except
      a. secondary sexual characteristics
      b. athletic ability
      c. functioning of accessory sex organs
      d. sex urges and behavior

34   6. The part of the sperm containing genes and chromosomes is called the

     ➤ a. head

        b. midsection

        c. tail

35   7. Cleavage begins to occur in the

        a. ovary   c. uterus prior to implantation

        b. fallopian tube   d. uterus after implantation

36–37   8. The blastoderm is composed of all of the following except

        a. ectoderm   c. mesoderm

        b. metroderm   d. endoderm

35   9. Cleavage is the process of cell division that takes place soon after

        a. menstruation   c. fertilization

        b. ovulation   d. implantation

FILL IN THE BLANK
Complete the following statements.

33   1. The time in the male's life when testosterone is first produced and secreted into the blood stream is called _Puberty_. *12–14*

35   2. When the head and neck of the sperm enter the ovum, the resulting cell is called a _fert – concept._

35   3. Soon after the nucleus of the sperm merges with the nucleus of the ovum, a series of cell divisions called _Cleavage_ begins. *36 h*

37   4. The cell nucleus of the human being contains _23_ pairs of chromosomes.

37–38   5. Human traits are determined through _genes_ that are found in _DNA_ .

37   6. Chromosomes are chains of giant molecules made up of _protein_ and _nucleic acid._

38   7. _____ *DNA* _____ contains the full genetic information of the human body and can be called the master template for cell building.

38   8. _____ *RNA* _____ is responsible for cell differentiation and is needed to make a bone cell different from a lung cell.

40   9. The incidence of fraternal twins depends upon _____ *race* _____,
_____ *humidity* _____, and _____ *age* _____ of the mother.

SHORT ANSWER

32   1. Explain how the male body regulates the temperature of sperm.

32   2. Why is the temperature of sperm important?

33   3. Where is the prostate gland located, and what is its function?

Surrounding urethra, and at base of bladder

milky secretion to semen
highly alkaline
stimulates sperm
action

38   4. What determines the sex of a baby?

38   5. Explain sex-linked characteristics, and list two examples:

Genes in X & Y

Hemophilia
Color Blindness *3 female*

39–40 6. Describe the genetic difference between identical twins and fraternal twins.

Same sex
I - Union of 1 sperm 1 ova
1 placenta 2 amniotic

Fr - 2 ova
2 sperms

2 amniotic sacs
Separate or fused placenta
1 out 250 births

23 & 40–42 7. Name three common reasons for infertility.

a._____

b._____

c._____

MATCHING

1. Match the terms in the left column with their definitions in the right column.

35	3	a. zygote	1.	early cell division
35	1	b. cleavage	2.	carries heredity elements
35	4	c. blastomeres	3.	sperm and ovum unite to form one cell with nucleus
37–38	2	d. chromosome	4.	produced by the first division of fertilized ovum
36	5	e. morula	5.	the mulberry appearance of a fertilized ovum after numerous cell divisions
36	6	f. blastocyst	6.	sphere of cells with hollow center that embeds in endometrium

36–37   2. The blastoderm is made up of distinct layers of cells that become the human system. Match the different layers to the anatomical parts they become.

2	a. endoderm	1.	brain, spinal cord, sensory organs, skin
3	b. mesoderm	2.	digestive tract lining stomach, liver, intestines
1	c. ectoderm	3.	skeleton, muscles, many internal organs

39   3. Label the following traits as dominant (D) or recessive (R).

D	a. dark hair		D	g. farsightedness
D	b. brown eyes		D	h. astigmatism
D	c. curly hair		D	i. glaucoma
R	d. blue eyes		R	j. myopia
R	e. light hair		R	k. diabetes mellitus
R	f. Rh-negative blood type		R	l. sickle cell anemia

EXERCISE

Mary and Peter have three sons and desperately want a daughter. Research the recommended methods to attempt to produce a female child.

CASE STUDY

Evelyn comes to the clinic in the eighth week of her first pregnancy. In taking the genetic history, it is learned that Evelyn's mother and her husband's father are affected with sickle cell anemia. Neither Evelyn nor her husband have any sign of the disease.

a. Is sickle cell anemia a dominant or recessive trait?

b. What counseling would the nurse give to Evelyn regarding the chances of having a child who develops sickle cell anemia?

CHAPTER

4

Fetal Development

MULTIPLE CHOICE
Select the one best answer.

49   1. The hormone in pregnancy that delays uterine contractions and helps to maintain the endometrium for continued fetal growth and development is

    a. estrogen

    b. progesterone

    c. human chorionic gonadotropin

    d. chorionic somatotrophin

52   2. The purpose of the amniotic fluid includes all of the following except to

    a. keep the fetus moist and maintain an even temperature

    b. cushion the fetus from injury

    c. equalize pressure around the fetus

    d. nourish the fetus

57   3. A cheese-like, greasy substance secreted by the sebaceous glands to protect the fetal skin is called

    a. decidua   c. vernix caseosa

    b. lanugo   d. subcutaneous fat

52   4. The short blood vessel between the pulmonary artery and the aorta of the fetus is called the

    a. ductus arteriosus   c. foramen ovale

    b. ductus venosus   d. inferior vena cava

52   5. The opening between the right and left auricles of the fetal heart is called the

    a. ductus arteriosus   c. foramen ovale

    b. ductus venosus   d. inferior vena cava

52   6. The fetal structure for passing fetal blood from the umbilical vein is called the
       a. ductus arteriosus   c. foramen ovale
       b. ductus venosus   d. inferior vena cava

54   7. The fertilized ovum is considered a fetus
       a. at conception
       b. with implantation
       c. when the first true bone replaces cartilage
       d. with recognized movement

48   8. Chorionic villi are fingerlike projections that
       a. develop from fetal tissue at the base of the implanted ovum
       b. become the afterbirth
       c. connect the cord to the placenta at the insertion site
       d. measures about 8 inches in diameter and weighs about ⅙ of baby's weight

49   9. The hormone that signals the corpus luteum to continue its stimulation of hormones
          to maintain the pregnancy is
       a. progesterone   c. chorionic somatotrophin
       b. estrogen   d. human chorionic gonadotropin

49   10. After the placenta has developed, the hormone(s) secreted to sustain the pregnancy
          include
       a. hCG and chorionic somatotrophin
       b. estrogen and progesterone
       c. progesterone
       d. gonadatropins

49   11. The hormone(s) produced by the placenta that are associated with fetal growth
          include
       a. progesterone
       b. estrogen and progesterone
       c. hCG and chorionic somatotrophin
       d. amniochorion

57   12. Meconium is composed of
       a. undigested food   c. bile, mucus, and epithelial cells
       b. digested food   d. bile and blood

FILL IN THE BLANK
Complete the following statements.

48   1. The portion of the endometrium that the ovum embeds into is
         called _uterine ceiling_.

48   2. Fingerlike projections that have developed from fetal tissue at the base of the
         implanted, fertilized ovum are called _Chorionic villi_.

49   3. The organ that acts as the respiratory, nutritive, and executory system for the fetus is
         called the _placenta_.

51   4. The "bag of waters" is composed of two membranes called _amnion_
         and _chorion_.

49   5. Nourishment passes from the maternal side of the placenta to the fetal side by the
         process of _osmosis_.

52   6. Too little amniotic fluid is termed _oligohydramnios_

52   7. As the blood flows from the ascending vena cava of the fetus into the auricle of the
         heart, it passes through the _foramen ovale_ directly into the
         left auricle.

52   8. Blood travels from the left auricle to the left ventricle and leaves the fetal heart
         through the _pulmonary artery_.

54   9. The umbilical vein in the baby's body becomes the _round lig. of liver_
         after delivery.

SHORT ANSWER

54   1. Name three structures that close and disappear after the baby is born.

         a. _____
         b. _____
         c. _____

57   2.   List four complications that can occur to the fetus or the pregnant woman when cocaine is used during pregnancy.

a. *Heart – tachycardia*

b. *Fetal activity*

c. *Abrupt uterine contractions*

d. *Preterm labor*

59–60   3.   List three diseases that can adversely affect the health of the fetus if contracted by the mother during pregnancy.

a. *Syphilis*   *Herpes simple*

b. *Gonorrhea*   *German Measles*

c. *Chlamydia*   *(rube*

CMC   *AIDS*

48   4.   Describe the umbilical cord, its vessels, and its function.

3 vessels   *2 to 4 ft*

Circulatory system between mother & fetus

to placenta

49   5.   Nourishing materials pass from the maternal side of the placenta to the fetal side by osmosis. Describe the process of osmosis.

less to more – equalizes

Semipermeable member

49   6.   Oxygen and carbon dioxide pass through the placenta by diffusion. Define diffusion.

permeable
2 gases at different concentrations
pass thru membrane
until equalized

53   7.   Trace the fetal circulation starting at the placenta.

48, 56   8.   Briefly describe the fetus as it develops through the 10 lunar months of pregnancy. Include approximate weight and length.

a. First month: _____

     Weight: _____ Length: _____

b. Second month: _____

     Weight: _____ Length: _____

c. Third month: _____

     Weight: _____ Length: _____

d. Fourth month: _____

     Weight: _____ Length: _____

e. Fifth month: _____

     Weight: _____ Length: _____

f. Sixth month: _____

     Weight: _____ Length: _____

g. Seventh month: _____

     Weight: _____ Length: _____

h. Eighth month: _____

     Weight: _____ Length: _____

i. Ninth month: _____

     Weight: _____ Length: _____

j. Tenth month: _____

     Weight: _____Length: _____

LABELING
Label the following diagram of fetal circulation.

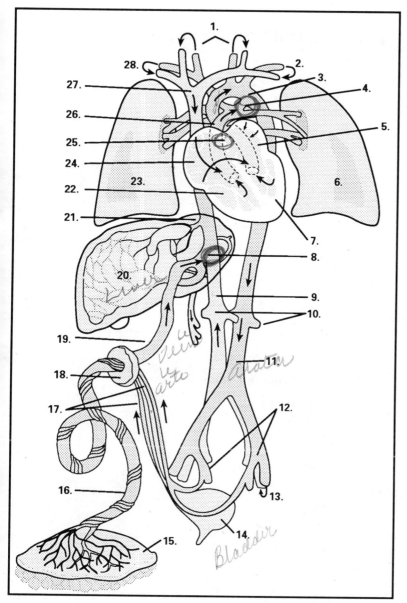

1._____

2._____

3._____

4._____

5._____

6._____

7._____

8._____

9._____

10._____

11._____

12._____

13._____

14._____

15._____

16._____

17._____

18._____

19._____

20._____

21._____

22._____

23._____

24._____

25._____

26._____

27._____

28._____

Signs and Symptoms of Pregnancy

MULTIPLE CHOICE

Select the one best answer.

73–74   1. A positive diagnosis of pregnancy can be made during the first six weeks with the aid of all of the following except

    a. hormone urine tests

    b. blood screen for hCG

    c. ultrasound

    d. blood test for progesterone level

68–69   2. The uterus grows from 2 ounces to _____during a pregnancy.

    a. 1 pound   c. ½ pound

    b. 2 pounds   d. 3 pounds

69   3. One of the most indicative signs of an early pregnancy on physical examination is

    a. chloasma

    b. striae

    c. softening of the lower portion of the uterus

    d. an enlarging uterus

69   4. The weight of the breasts increases during pregnancy due to

    a. milk production

    b. increased fatty deposits

    c. colostrum production

    d. increased glandular tissue and blood supply

69   5. The pelvis spreads out slightly during pregnancy for all the following reasons except
     a.   pressure of the baby
     b.   change in posture
     c.   relaxation of muscles
     d.   hormonal changes

69   6. The mask of pregnancy is also called
     a.   chloasma   c.   Chadwick's sign
     b.   linea nigra   d.   Goodell's sign

70   7. Blood volume increase reaches its peak during the
     a.   third month of pregnancy
     b.   fifth month of pregnancy
     c.   seventh month of pregnancy   *7-8 month*
     d.   last weeks of pregnancy

70   8. Varicose veins are common in pregnancy and are found in all of the following areas except the
     a.   abdomen   c.   rectum
     b.   vulva   d.   legs

70   9. Cystitis can occur in pregnancy due to all of the following except
     a.   dilated ureters caused by the growing uterus exerting pressure on the ureters as they cross the pelvic brim
     b.   the softening of the ureteral walls as a result of endocrine influences
     c.   the loss of ureteral muscle tone making it more difficult to expel urine
     d.   the weight the fetus exerts downward on the bladder causing frequency of urination

71   10. Digestive changes that commonly occur during pregnancy include all of the following except
     a.   nausea   c.   constipation
     b.   appetite changes   d.   irritable bowel syndrome

71   11. The anterior lobe of the pituitary gland secretes hormones that act on all of the following except
     a.   uterus   c.   thyroid
     b.   ovaries   d.   breasts

72   12. Chadwick's sign appears around the   *1st trimester*
     a.   eighth week of pregnancy
     b.   second week of pregnancy
     c.   fourth week of pregnancy
     d.   first week after implantation

73   13. Micturition is defined as

        a. painful urination

        b. pressure with urination

        (c.) frequency of urination

        d. blood detected in the urine

73   14. Quickening can usually by felt by the mother and the care provider by the

        a. 16th week   c. 18th week

        b. 24th week   (d.) 20th week

74   15. With the use of ultrasound, an intrauterine pregnancy can usually be confirmed by the

        (a.) fourth to the sixth week of pregnancy

        b. second to the fourth week of pregnancy

        c. sixth to the eighth week of pregnancy

        d. tenth week of pregnancy

FILL IN THE BLANK
Complete the following statements.

67   1. The uterus eventually increases ___500 %___ times larger than its original size by the end of the pregnancy.

71   2. The recommended weight gain during pregnancy is ___25 – 30___ pounds.

70   3. During a pregnancy, the urinary system changes with the amount of urine ___↑___ and the specific gravity ___∨___ .

71   4. The hormone released from the posterior lobe of the pituitary gland that stimulates uterine contractions is called ___oxytocin___ .

74   5. The funic souffle is a soft murmur produced by ___umbilical arteries___ .

SHORT ANSWER

69   1. Describe how the mother's muscular and skeletal systems change during pregnancy.

Muscle tone loss
Muscle fibers↑
Skeletal greater blood supply in bone
marrow.

69–70   2. Describe circulatory changes in the mother's body during pregnancy.

70   3. Name three signs of preeclampsia.
   a. _____ hypertension _____
   b. _____ edem _____
   c. _____ albuminuria _____

71   4. List the eight changes in the pregnant woman that account for her weight gain, and give the approximate weight gain expected for each.

a.	Fetus	7½ pounds
b.	Placenta	1 pounds
c.	Amniotic fluid	2 pounds
d.	Uterus	2 pounds
e.	Breasts	1½ pounds
f.	Blood volume	2½ pounds
g.	Fat	5 pounds
h.	Tissue fluid	6 pounds

27½

72–73 5. Name seven presumptive signs of pregnancy.

   a. _linea nigra_
   b. _areola of breast_
   c. _Chadwick sign_
   d. _Amenorrhea_
   e. _nausea/vomiting_
   f. _freq. urination_
   g. _Chloasma_

73 6. Name five probable signs of pregnancy.

   a. _Chang in abd_   d. _Ballottement_
   b. _Hegar_   e. _Braxton-_
   c. _Goodell_   _Hick sig_

74 7. Name five positive signs of pregnancy.

   a. _Fetal HR_   d. _funic souffle_
   b. _movement_   e. _placental souffle_
   c. _Ultrasound_
      X ray

69 8. State the purpose of Braxton-Hicks contractions.

   Painless intermittent contractions
   uterus enlarges to accommodate
   growing fetus & developing power
   to expel baby

69 9. List three skin changes that commonly occur in pregnancy.

   a. _linea nigra_
   b. _Chloasma_
   c. _striae gravidarum_

70 10. Briefly explain why it is normal for a pregnant woman's hemoglobin to be slightly lower than in a nonpregnant state.

   Increase of fluid

71   11. A woman who suffers from heartburn during her pregnancy should be instructed to

     a. _small meals_____

     b. _✓ fat_____

     c. _lessen worries_____

69   12. Striae gravidarum is caused by

     _Stretching of skin_____

_____

73   13. A positive urine pregnancy test is considered a probable sign of pregnancy, not a positive sign because

     _Misinterpreting_____

     _Not following directions_____

_____

_____

MATCHING

67   1. Match the terms in the left column with their definitions in the right column.

     __4__ a. primipara   1. woman pregnant with her first child

     __3__ b. nullipara   2. woman who has been pregnant several times

     __2__ c. multigravida   3. woman who has not borne children

     __5__ d. multipara   4. woman in labor with or having borne her first child

     __1__ e. primigravida   5. woman in labor with, or having borne, her second or subsequent child

72–73   2. Match the following signs of pregnancy with their definitions.

     __3__ a. Hegar's sign   1. softening of the cervix

     __1__ b. Goodell's sign   2. intermittent painless contractions

     __4__ c. Chadwick's sign   3. softening of lower portion of the uterus

     __2__ d. Braxton-Hicks   4. bluish-purple color of vaginal tissue

     __5__ e. ballottement   5. rebounding of the fetus on exam

3. Match the following skin changes with their definitions.

a. __3__ striae gravidarum

1. dark line from umbilicus to mons pubis

b. __1__ linea nigra

2. freckle-like pigmentation on the face

c. __2__ chloasma

3. red streaks on the abdomen, breasts, or thighs caused by skin stretching

CASE STUDIES

1. Ann, a 23-year-old woman, enters the clinic complaining of amenorrhea, tender breasts, excessive fatigue, and frequent urination. She also states she is nauseated and feels like she must have the flu.

   a. What tests should the nurse perform?

   b. What questions should the nurse ask to help determine a diagnosis?

2. Betty visits the clinic for her regular prenatal appointment. She is a 28-year-old woman in the 26th week of her first pregnancy. Betty states she drank 50 gm of Glucola approximately one hour ago, as instructed, to be screened for gestational diabetes. Her weight gain was 1.5 pounds during the past month. Her urine is negative for protein but positive for glucose. Her blood pressure is 110/64. FHT are strong and approximately 148 beats per minute. Betty is complaining of a bad headache that just "came on." What can the nurse tell Betty about her headache, about her weight gain, about her urine test, about her blood pressure, and about the baby's heart beat?

CHAPTER 6

Nursing Care and Medical Supervision

MULTIPLE CHOICE
Select the one best answer.

83   1. A woman with a confirmed positive pregnancy should start receiving prenatal care
   a. in the third month of pregnancy
   b. as soon as she has missed a period
   c. as soon as she has missed two periods
   d. when she feels movement

84   2. Which of the following is *not* a part of the health history?
   a. allergies
   b. contraceptive use
   c. past pregnancies and their outcomes
   d. date of most recent coitus

90   3. The condition in which the fetus has retarded growth, neurological abnormalities, microcephaly, microphthalmia, and a poorly developed philtrum is
   a. neural tube defect
   b. cocaine addicted syndrome
   c. fetal alcohol syndrome
   d. Down syndrome

91   4. The effects of smoking on the fetus include all but
   a. lower birth weight at term and greater chance of premature birth
   b. greater risk of perinatal death
   c. placenta abnormalities
   d. delayed brain cell development

5. Information gathered from various family members for the nursing care process is considered

    a. subjective information

    b. objective information

    c. informal information

    d. not appropriate information to include in plan

6. Information gathered by direct observation is considered

    a. subjective information

    b. objective information

    c. formal information

    d. primary basis for assessment

7. Implementation of a nursing care plan includes all of the following except

    a. performing a nursing procedure

    b. offering physical or emotional support

    c. counseling or instructing

    d. explaining the plan to the health team

8. Anemia in pregnancy is defined as a hemoglobin level of less than

    a. 8 g/dL   c. 12 g/dL

    b. 10 g/dL   d. 14 g/dL

9. Iron deficiency anemia occurs in pregnancy because of all the following except

    a. the amount of iron required exceeds what is provided by maternal stores

    b. the absorption of iron from the maternal gastrointestinal tract is decreased

    c. the fetus demands a high level of iron throughout the entire pregnancy

    d. the woman may not be eating a proper diet or taking her prenatal vitamins

10. Advice regarding over-the-counter medications should include:

    a. It is acceptable to take OTC medication for symptomatic relief of various problems in the middle trimester only.

    b. It is acceptable to take OTC medication after the 12th week of pregnancy.

    c. All medication should have prior physician approval.

    d. Medication should be avoided throughout the entire pregnancy unless absolutely necessary.

86–87   11. The maternal serum alphafetoprotein level is measured
      a. between the 10th and 12th week gestation
      b. between the 15th and 20th week gestation   *p. 160*
      c. between the 26th and 28th week gestation
      d. before the 12th week gestation

87   12. An increased level of AFP suggests
      a. spina bifida or anencephaly
      b. meningitis
      c. Down syndrome
      d. blood incompatibility

87   13. Gestational diabetes is screened
      a. in the 21st week gestation
      b. in the 18th week gestation
      c. between the 24th and 26th week gestation
      d. between the 20th and 24th week gestation

90   14. Aspirin taken in pregnancy can
      a. cause no harm
      b. prolong bleeding time
      c. cause skeletal anomalies
      d. cause fetal kidney damage

90   15. Alcohol consumed during pregnancy can cause all of the following except
      a. the alteration of embryonic organization of tissue
      b. the interference with carbohydrate, lipid, and protein metabolism
      c. an affect on the fetal central nervous system
      d. an affect on the fetal liver

FILL IN THE BLANK
Complete the following statements.

88   1. At 28 weeks' gestation, the fundal height would be expected to measure
      _____28_____ cm.

78   2. Care of the pregnant woman before her delivery is called prenatal or
      _____antepartum_____care.

87   3. A serum Glucola level of over ___*140*___ mg/dL would suggest gestational diabetes, and further testing would be indicated.

91   4. Three commonly consumed products that are high in caffeine include ___*Coffee*___, ___*tea*___, and ___*Cocoa*___.

78   5. Three ways to obtain the information needed to formulate a care plan include ___*(Assess) direct obser.*___, ___*Interview*___, and ___*exam*___.

87   6. The blood test to screen for neural tube defects is called ___*AFP*___.

160   7. The blood test to help screen for Down syndrome is called ___*AFP*___.

SHORT ANSWER

78–80 1. What are the four separate steps in the nursing care process?

a. ___*Assess*___

b. ___*Plan*___

c. ___*Implementation*___

d. ___*Evaluation*___

79   2. Explain the difference between objective and subjective information.

79   3. List three purposes of a nursing care plan.

plan
implement
evaluate

a. ___*Identify*___

b. ___*organize*___   *problems*

c. ___*documenting*___   *of pt*

80–81   4. Define the medical SOAP method for care plans.

    a. S: _Subj_____

    b. O: _Obj'_____

    c. A: _assess_____

    d. P: _plan_____

85   5. Name four questions a woman should be asked about her menstruation in obtaining a history.

    a. _When did she start mense_____

    b. _Regular periods? – painful_____

    c. _How long?_____

    d. _1st day of last period_____

85   6. Explain Naegle's rule for determining the estimated date of delivery.

86   7. Name four purposes for the internal pelvic examination of the pregnant woman.

    a. _Pap smear – cervical smear_____

    b. _Exam vagina + pelvic for signs of preg._

    c. _Abnormalities – cysts or infection_____

    d. _Determine true pelvis to pass baby_____

86   8. List four lab tests routinely performed on the pregnant woman at her first exam.

    a. _Urine (sugar, albumen, nitrites, leukocytes_

AFP   b. _Blood (hepatitis, bloodtype, Rh factor, rubella_

                                      Syphilis

    c. _Diabetes_____

    d. _Gr. B streptococci_____

        AFP

89   9. List four things the nurse should discuss with the expectant mother regarding planning for the baby.

    a. _Who will provide health care for baby___

    b. _Breast or Bottle_____

    c. _If male – circumcision_____

    d. _What do you know about care of_____
       baby

89   10. Name eight danger signals in pregnancy.

a. _____

b. _____

c. _____

d. _____

e. _____

f. _____

g. _____

h. _____

79   11. Place the following basic human needs described by Maslow in order of priority.

3 2 love and belonging

4 #1 self-actualization

1 4 physiological needs ← *bottom level God air sex food*

2 3 safety and security

80   12. When asking a patient to describe her symptoms, name at least six specific descriptive terms that should be explored about the disorder.

a. *onset*   d. *radiation*

b. *character*   e. *duration*

c. *location*   f. *frequency*

82   13. List three objective signs of iron deficiency.

a. *Pallor*

b. *tachycardia*

c. *Hemoglobin > 10.0 g/dL   hematocrit 7 31%*

83   14. State the meaning of the acronym TPAL.

a. T: *term*

b. P: *premature*

c. A: *abortions*

d. L: *living*

85   15. Ana's LMP was 2–10–93. It was normal in flow and duration. No contraceptives were being used. She has 28-day menstrual cycles. What was the probable date of conception? What is the expected date of delivery?

a. _____

b. _____

86   16. Define the lithotomy position.

Supine c feet in stirrup
butt at end of table

88   17. Name five things that are examined at each return visit to the physician's office during a pregnancy.

a. _BP & wt_

b. _Urine_

c. _Abdomen_

d. _fetal heartbeat 130/160_

e. _Pelvic exam_

88   18. The height of the uterine fundus can be measured or estimated to help determine appropriate fetal growth. Name the expected anatomical landmarks where the fundus might be found at each of the following weeks' gestation.

a.   12 weeks   _top of symphsis_

b.   16 weeks   _midway between symphsis & umbilicus_

c.   20 weeks   _umbilicus_

d.   36 weeks   _xiphoid_

88   19. Briefly describe Leopold's maneuvers.

Outline of fetus is determined
by palpation along sides

91   20. List three dangers of smoking to the expectant mother and her fetus.

Fetus   Mother

a. _↓ placenta blood flow_   _lung cancer_

b. _premature birth_   _vascular disease_   91

c. _perinatal_   _cardiac_
     death

91   21. Briefly describe how caffeine affects the system and a pregnancy.

↑ production
of epinephrine
& norepinephrine

MATCHING

Match the following drug categories with their correct FDA classification.

_____2___ a. animal studies have not disclosed any fetal risk, but no
           adequate human studies are available   1. A

_____5___ b. contraindicated during pregnancy   2. B

_____1___ c. well-controlled human studies show no fetal risk   3. C

_____3___ d. animal studies reveal some fetal effects, but no   4. D

          human studies are available   5. X

_____4___ e. some fetal risk, but benefits outweigh the risks

CASE STUDIES

1. Lori is a 23-year-old woman, pregnant with her first baby. She was the youngest child in her family and feels she knows nothing about pregnancy and becoming a parent. She is happily married and is excited about this pregnancy. She states she is in good health. What information does the nurse need to get from Lori, and what information should she give Lori in this initial visit for her pregnancy?

2. Elizabeth is a pregnant woman seeking prenatal care for the first time at 24 weeks' gestation. She is a gravida 3, para 0, and is 22 years old. She is on welfare, unmarried, and has no family in the area. She lives in low-cost housing and is looking for work. She has not graduated from high school. She smokes a pack of cigarettes a day, and her diet is poor. The father of the baby is her current boyfriend, but they have no marriage plans. He is also unemployed. Design a nursing care plan. Choose at least two physical and two social issues as a basis for your plan of care.

CHAPTER 7

Normal Pregnancy

MULTIPLE CHOICE

Select the one best answer.

97
1. Constipation may be a problem during pregnancy for all of the following reasons except
   a. decreased physical exertion
   b. relaxation of smooth muscle
   c. obstruction of the lower bowel by the fetus
   d. increase in milk consumption

97
2. A strong odor in the urine during the first trimester of pregnancy indicates
   a. not enough fluid intake
   b. excreted hormones
   c. infection
   d. stress on the kidneys

99
3. The purpose of strengthening pelvic floor muscles during pregnancy includes all of the following except to
   a. decrease constipation
   b. help support the uterus and bladder
   c. help push effectively at the time of delivery
   d. decrease involuntary loss of urine

116
4. Pressure of the fetus exerted downward in the pelvis is, in part, the cause of all of the following discomforts except
   a. flatulence and back ache
   b. hemorrhoids and varicose veins
   c. swelling feet
   d. insomnia

96   5. The advice the nurse should give about bathing during pregnancy includes
    a. don't take a tub bath
    b. don't use soap because it is drying
    c. daily bathing or showering is recommended
    d. bath water can enter the vagina and carry infection to the uterus

97   6. A pregnant woman who complains of constipation should be advised to
    a. take a mild laxative
    b. increase water and fiber in her diet
    c. exercise more vigorously
    d. use an enema

100   7. An exercise program acceptable during pregnancy includes
    a. housework, walking, and mild recreation
    b. snow and water skiing in the early months
    c. horseback riding
    d. high impact aerobics

101   8. Protein demands increase during pregnancy from the RDA recommended 46 gm/day to
    a. 76 gm/day   c. 65 gm/day
    b. 60 gm/day   d. 58 gm/day

101   9. Iron requirements during pregnancy increase from 15 mg/day (RDA) to
    a. 45 mg/day   c. 30 mg/day
    b. 20 mg/day   d. 60 mg/day

103   10. Citrus fruits are the best sources of vitamin C and also have
    a. vitamin D   c. vitamin E
    b. vitamins A and B   d. iron

104   11. The main value of meat is the
    a. protein it provides   c. amino acids it provides
    b. iron it provides   d. calories it supplies

106–107 12. Common discomforts in pregnancy include all of the following except
    a. bleeding gums and nose bleeds
    b. itching skin
    c. excessive thirst
    d. increased vaginal discharge

126   13. Having many children is viewed as a social service and a rewarded event for women who live in

- (a.) France   c. Italy
- b. Germany   d. Russia

127–128   14. Joseph DeLee was an obstetrician who in 1920 recommended the routine use of

- a. medication during labor
- b. fetal monitoring during labor
- (c.) forceps, episiotomy, and early removal of the placenta
- d. delivering breech positioned babies by Cesarean section

129   15. The unmarried, newly delivered mother should be

- a. encouraged to give her baby up for adoption
- b. put in a private room for her postpartum experience and treated with sympathy
- (c.) encouraged to express any concerns and be supported in her new role
- d. informed about the emotional and financial support the newborn will need through life

FILL IN THE BLANK

99   1 The exercise to help tone the pelvic floor muscles is called the _____*Kegel*_____ exercise.

100   2. The American College of Obstetrics and Gynecology recommends a woman's heart rate not exceed ____*140*____ beats per minute during exercise.

101   3. During a pregnancy, a woman will need an additional ____*300*____ calories a day to maintain health and nutritionally support her fetus.

105   4. The recommended weight gain range is ____*25 – 30*____ pounds by the end of her pregnancy.

111   5. A process whereby the mother is conditioned to control the pain of childbirth through information, breathing, and relaxation exercises is called ____*natural childbirth*____ *(3)*

101   6. An inadequate amount of protein in the pregnant woman's diet may affect the quantity of ____*brain cells*____ in the fetus.

102–103   7. The vitamin and mineral content in fresh vegetables can be destroyed by

_____*cooking*_____ .

SHORT ANSWER

96   1. Name three suggestions that might help chronic backache during pregnancy.

a. *Exercise*

b. *Proper shoes*

c. *Good posture & body alignment*

111   2. List four benefits of childbirth preparation classes.

a. *Less anxious*

b. *Information — factual preg. labor & delivery*

c. *Physical condition*

d. *Information about breast, postpartum & infant care*

97   3. If, during the physical exam, it is noted that the pregnant woman has inverted nipples, she should be instructed to

Massage gently

99–100   4. List three benefits of the perineal squeeze.

a. *Helps avoid involuntary loss of urine*

b. *Help support the uterus & bladder in proper position*

c. *Will aid pushing out the baby.*

100–101   5. If a woman plans to travel at any time during her pregnancy, she should be advised to

Walk, after a few hours of sitting

Why? *Prevent slow down of her circulation*

96   6. Stockings with elastic tops should be avoided during pregnancy because

_____

103–104   7. Name three benefits of dairy foods in pregnancy.

a. *Calcium*

b. *phosphorus*

c. *Vit A*

104–105 8. If a pregnant woman is a vegetarian, what foods can the nurse suggest that will supply the essential nutrients of meat?

Legumes & Veg

105 9. Define pica.

hunger for non food – clay

113 10. Limiting food to small amounts frequently may help decrease nausea in pregnancy because

Slows gastric motility in preg. patients

118 11. List four causes of swelling in the feet.
   a. _Na_
   b. _↑ venous pressure_
   c. _↑ capillary permeability_
   d. _dietary protein deficiency_

118 12. Name three reasons for leg cramps during pregnancy.
   a. _lg amt of milk_
   b. _fatigue_
   c. _Sudden stretching of leg & foot_

120 13. List the most likely causes of fainting and dizziness during pregnancy.
   a. _hypoglycemia_
   b. _hyperventilation_
   c. _Anemia_
   d. _Sudden movement_

124 14. List four possible influences thought to be responsible for mood swings during pregnancy.
   a. _hormonal changes_
   b. _inadg rest_
   c. _" " diet_
   d. _feelings of preg._

111 15. Describe the basic principles taught in childbirth preparation classes.
   a. _Intellectual_
   b. _Physical_
   c. _Exercise training & breathing_

111   16. Define psychoprophylaxis.   *P. 111*

       Lamaze

_____

_____

_____

127–128   17. Name three areas of management during labor that vary from one culture to another.

      a. *medicine* _____

      b. *Birthing positions* _____

      c. *Coach* _____

128   18. Why is it important for the nurse to recognize different cultural practices?

MATCHING

1.   Match the food or nutrient with the appropriate function.

Page	Answer		Food/Nutrient		Function
104	*1*	a.	breads and cereals	1.	can act as laxative
103	*3*	b.	milk	2.	increases resistance to infection
103	*2*	c.	vitamin A	3.	supplies high levels of calcium and phosphorus
102–103	*6*	d.	vegetables	4.	cannot be stored
104	*5*	e.	meat	5.	amino acid source
104–105	*7*	f.	dried beans, peas, and nuts	6.	provides carbohydrates thiamine, riboflavin, and niacin
102	*4*	g.	vitamin C	7.	meat substitute

2. Match the culture with the correct tradition.

126	_____	a. African
126	_____	b. Canadian Eskimo
126	_____	c. American
126	_____	d. French
126	_____	e. Swedish
128	_____	f. Goajiro Indian
128	_____	g. Philippine

1. Childbirth is viewed as a medical event.

2. The spirit enters the baby in early pregnancy.

3. The father's clan spirit enters the baby in early pregnancy, and the mother's clan spirit enters after birth.

4. Childbirth is viewed as a fulfilling personal achievement.

5. Official state policy encourages women to have as many babies as possible.

6. Eating a bird will keep the baby small, and eating an octopus can make the fetus stick inside the mother.

7. Newly delivered women stay in bed for up to a month.

3. Match the following elements to their function. There may be more than one answer for some elements.

108	___/___ 5	a. calcium
108	__7__ 2	b. zinc
108	___|___	c. phosphorus
108	__6__	d. iron
108	__8__	e. iodine
107	__3__	f. protein
108	_____	g. magnesium
109	___/___	h. vitamin A
109	__5__	i. vitamin K
110	_____	j. vitamin C

1. helps build bone and teeth

2. important growth of nervous system

3. builds and repairs tissues

4. helps form antibodies

5. important in blood clotting

6. combines with protein to make hemoglobin

7. component of insulin

8. controls the rate of body's energy use

EXERCISE

Research and write a paper on the childbirth practices of a different culture. Include antepartal care, labor and delivery choices, postpartum recovery, and early infant care practices.

CHAPTER

8

Complications of Pregnancy

MULTIPLE CHOICE
Select the one best answer.

139   1. PIH (pregnancy induced hypertension) is defined as a blood
        pressure above
        a.   130/80   c.   140/90
        b.   150/100   d.   140/100

151   2. A vaginal discharge that produces a fish odor is
        a.   trichomonas   c.   chlamydia
        b.   bacterial vaginosis d.   candidiasis

141   3. Placenta abruptio is usually
        a.   painful
        b.   painless

139   4. The delivery of choice for a woman with a partial placenta
        previa is
        a.   vaginal delivery
        b.   cesarean section

155   5. An intrauterine transfusion is the injection of Rh negative
        erythrocytes into the
        a.   peritoneal cavity of the fetus
        b.   amniotic fluid
        c.   umbilical vein
        d.   mother's blood stream

135   6. All the following are danger signs of pregnancy except
        a.   severe continuous headaches
        b.   chills and fever
        c.   swelling of feet at the end of the day
        d.   persistent nausea or vomiting

47

135   7. Pain in the abdomen or back during pregnancy may be a sign of any of the following except

     a. ectopic pregnancy

     b. placenta abruptio

     c. preterm labor contractions

     d. preeclampsia

135   8. An ectopic pregnancy is usually found in

     a. the abdomen   c. the ovary

     b. the fallopian tube   d. the uterus

136   9. A hydatidiform mole is

     a. an uncommon occurrence

     b. a fairly common occurrence

     c. more common with women over 30 years of age

     d. more common in teens

136   10. The follow-up care for hydatidiform mole is important because of the risk of

     a. a future miscarriage

     b. malignant chorion carcinoma

     c. excessive bleeding

     d. a repeated molar pregnancy

137   11. A missed abortion is one in which

     a. part of the product of conception is passed, but part remains in the uterus

     b. the fetus dies in utero, but the product of conception is retained

     c. the entire product of conception is expelled without the aid of a D&C

     d. an incomplete D&C is performed for a desired termination of pregnancy

135   12. If a woman presents with a positive pregnancy test and is having bleeding and cramping, the care provider should

     a. suspect an ectopic pregnancy or a miscarriage

     b. assume this is normal

     c. wait and watch to see if miscarriage occurs

     d. schedule a D&C

138   13. Twins occur in pregnancy at a rate of

     a. 1:800 pregnancies   c. 1:80 pregnancies

     b. 1:6400 pregnancies   d. 1:200 pregnancies

138 14. Complications more common in multiple pregnancies than in singleton pregnancies include all of the following except

    a. PIH   c. low birth weight babies

    b. premature labor   d. miscarriage

138 15. Hyperemesis gravidarum will be evident by all the following symptoms except

    a. pitting edema   c. dehydration

    b. nausea   d. weight loss

139 16. When a pregnant woman is experiencing symptoms of preeclampsia, her urine

    a. output may be decreased

    b. output may be increased

    c. may have bacteria

    d. may test positive for glucose and nitrites

139 17. The distinguishing characteristic(s) between preeclampsia and eclampsia is/are

    a. convulsions   c. visual changes and hyperactive reflexes

    b. higher blood pressure   d. edema

139 18. Preeclampsia occurs more often in all of the following except

    a. women under 15 years or over 35 years old

    b. nutritionally deficient women

    c. diabetic women

    d. multigravida women

139 19. The risks of placenta previa include all of the following except

    a. bleeding   c. infection

    b. shock   d. preterm laborn

142 20. Some women develop gestational diabetes because of all the following reasons except

    a. the fetus grows rapidly during the last trimester

    b. the placenta and the mother's body produce substances that raise the mother's blood sugar

    c. the pancreas is unable to make enough extra insulin

    d. the woman consumes too much sugar

142 21. Diabetic women have an increased incidence of all of the following complications except

    a. abortions

    b. stillbirths and premature labor

    c. congenital defects in the newborn

    d. low birth weight babies

144   22. Infants delivered at term to diabetic women have a higher mortality rate than those delivered earlier because of

    a. a hypoglycemic reaction

    b. vascular changes in the placenta

    c. maternal hypertension

    d. liver damage

146   23. Women who have a greater tendency to develop gestational diabetes include all of the following except

    a. obese women

    b. women with a family history of diabetes

    c. women who consume large quantities of sugar

    d. women under severe emotional stress

147   24. Bacterial vaginosis has also been called all of the following except

    a. hemophilus   c. *Gardnerella*

    b. candidiasis   d. nonspecific vaginitis

148   25. Genital warts are medically termed

    a. *Trichomonas vaginalis*   c. condylomata acuminato

    b. leukorrhea   d. chlamydia

150–151   26. An infectious disease that may affect the heart, long bones, skin, and respiratory system of the fetus is

    a. AIDS   c. syphilis

    b. chlamydia   d. gonorrhea

151   27. The infectious, sexually transmitted disease of which 60%-80% of infected women will not have symptoms is

    a. chlamydia   c. gonorrhea

    b. syphilis   d. condylomata acuminato

152   28. Which of the following statements about HIV is *not* correct?

    a. A large percentage of people exposed to HIV may never develop the physical symptoms of immune suppression.

    b. Many people infected with HIV have no symptoms and feel well.

    c. People with a positive HIV test are infectious and can pass the virus to others even if they have no symptoms.

    d. HIV is characterized by fever, fatigue, loss of appetite and weight, night sweats, unexplained diarrhea, swollen glands, a dry cough, and unexplained skin lesions.

153   29. A disease that, if contracted in the first three months of pregnancy, can cause
        cataracts, heart lesions, deaf-mutism, and microcephaly is
        a. fifth disease   c. scarlet fever
        b. rubella   d. rubeola

153–154 30. All of the following statements are true about fifth disease except:
        a. If infection occurs in latter pregnancy, it can cause preterm labor. *anemia*
        b. It is caused by human parvovirus.
        c. If infection occurs in early pregnancy, it can cause miscarriage.
        d. It causes flu-like illness with a rash.

154   31. RhoGAM is a medication given
        a. to women whose partners have Rh-negative blood
        b. to women who have Rh-negative blood
        c. only to women who are Rh-negative and carrying an Rh-positive baby
        d. only to women who are Rh-positive and carrying an Rh-negative baby

154   32. Erythroblastosis fetalis is a hemolytic disease of the newborn characterized by all of
        the following symptoms except
        a. anemia
        b. jaundice and liver enlargement
        c. heart failure and brain damage if severe
        d. respiratory problems

FILL IN THE BLANK
Complete the following statements.

135   1. A pregnancy located outside of the uterus is called an _____ pregnancy.

135   2. A pregnancy in which the fertilized ovum degenerates and the chorionic villi convert
        into a mass of transparent cysts is called a _____ pregnancy.

136   3. The hormone ___hCG___ is followed closely after a
        molar pregnancy is terminated.

138   4. When two or more embryos develop in the uterus at the same time, it is termed
        _____ pregnancy.

147   5. High levels of ketones in the urine is a sign that the body has switched to burning
        ___fat___ for energy and can be harmful to the fetus.

149 6. If a newborn passes through a birth canal infected with *Neisseria gonorrheae*, it is at

risk for _____ *blindness / eye infection*

154 7. _____ *RhoGam* is given to Rh-negative women shortly after delivery

of an Rh-positive baby to prevent the formation of antibodies.

154 8. The hemolytic condition in which antibodies from an Rh-negative mother react

against the Rh-positive infant is called _____ *Erythroblastosis feta*

139 9. Preeclampsia rarely occurs before the _____ *24th* _____ week of pregnancy.

154 10. If a woman is exposed to fifth disease in the first trimester or early second trimester

of pregnancy, she is at an increased risk for *miscarriage* _____ .

SHORT ANSWER

136 1. List three symptoms that suggest a molar pregnancy.

   a. *bleeding* _____ *passage of grape*
   b. *nausea* _____ *like vessels*
   c. *absent of fetal heart tone*
   PID

138 2. Name three signs that might suggest a multiple pregnancy.

   a. *2 HB heard*
   b. *family history*
   c. *wt gain is rapid*

138 3. List two possible complications that may occur in multiple pregnancy.

   a. *Hypertension*
   b. *Prematurity*

139 4. Name five signs of preeclampsia.

   a. *albuminuria*
   b. *Hypertension*
   c. *Edema*
   d. *rapid wt gain*
   e. *reflexes maybe*
   hyperactive

141–142   5.   Gestational diabetes is screened at the end of the second trimester. Why?

Growth of fetus

142–143   6.   Why do gestationally diabetic women have more urinary tract infections?

because the presence of sugar in the urine favors growth of bacteria

142–144   7.   Name three possible complications that might occur in the gestationally diabetic woman.

    a.   *large fetus / cong. defects*
    b.   *premature labor / abortion*
    c.   *hydramnios   preclampsia*

146   8.   List three common symptoms of diabetes.

    a.   *thirst*
    b.   *hunger*
    c.   *freq. urine*

147   9.   What symptom is the most prominent when a woman has vaginal candidiasis?

Edema of external genitals
itching
cheesy discharge

152   10. List three ways HIV is transmitted.

a. _____

b. _____

c. _____

153   11. Name six CDC precautions to be followed by all health professionals to avoid becoming infected with HIV.

a. _____

b. _____

c. _____

d. _____

e. _____

f. _____

154   12. Toxoplasmosis is a parasite and can infect humans by

a. *animals*

b. *raw / uncooked meat*

139   13. List the meaning of the HELLP blood screen to evaluate preeclampsia.

a. H: *hemolysis*

b. E: *elevated*

c. L: *liver enzymes*

d. L: *low*

e. P: *platelets*

MATCHING

137   Match the terms in the left column with their definitions in the right column.

_1_   a. spontaneous abortion   1. termination of pregnancy through natural causes

_4_   b. induced abortion   2. the entire product of conception is expelled spontaneously

_2_   c. complete abortion   3. part of the product of conception is expelled, and some remains in the uterus

_3_   d. incomplete abortion   4. termination of pregnancy with the aid of mechanical means

_5_   e. missed abortion   5. the fetus dies in utero, but the product of conception is retained

CASE STUDIES

1. Becky is a 37-year-old primipara who comes in for a routine office visit at 36 weeks' gestation. The nurse finds Becky's blood pressure at 150/94. She also notes a weight gain of 8 pounds since her last visit 2 weeks ago. Becky's urine has 2+ protein, negative sugar, and negative nitrites. Create a nursing care plan for Becky.

2. Sue is a 32-year-old pregnant woman in her 28th week of pregnancy. She has a history of gestational diabetes in her previous pregnancy. What are the important questions to ask and tests to perform at this office visit? Discuss indications for follow-up depending on your findings. Review the impact of gestational diabetes.

Assessing Fetal Well-Being

MULTIPLE CHOICE
Select the one best answer.

160   1. AFP (alphafetoprotein) measurement is used prenatally to screen for
    a. lung maturity
    b. neural tube defects
    c. diabetes
    d. blood incompatibility

160   2. The AFP measurement is most accurate if drawn between _____weeks of pregnancy.
    a. 13–16   c. 24–26
    b. 15–20   d. 26–28

160   3. The AFP value can be falsely abnormal for all of the following reasons except
    a. incorrect dates
    b. the woman has gestational diabetes
    c. lab error
    d. multiple pregnancy

160   4. The triple screen (AFP, hCG, and estriol level) is a test for
    a. neural tube defects
    b. anencephaly
    c. Down syndrome
    d. hydrocephaly

162   5. Amniocentesis is performed for genetic testing between the _____weeks of pregnancy.
    a. 6–13   c. 18–24
    b. 15–18   d. 20–22

166–167   6. A nonstress test is performed to
    a. check for fetal maturity
    b. check for fetal well-being
    c. check the mother's blood pressure reaction with uterine contractions
    d. check mother's perception of fetal movement

165   7. In ultrasound, white reflections indicate fetal
    a. tissue   c. muscle
    b. fluids   d. bone

165   8. The test most commonly performed to determine fetal age when dating is uncertain is
    a. the pelvic exam   c. ultrasound
    b. amniocentesis   d. hCG levels

166   9. The 24-hour urinary estrogen is measured to assess
    a. placental functioning   c. fetal lung maturity
    b. fetal liver maturity   d. gestational diabetes

166   10. A biophysical profile score considered to demonstrate fetal well-being is
    a. >8   c. >6
    b. >10   d. >5

162   11. The lecithin-sphingomyelin (LS) ratio measures
    a. lung surfactant phospholipids and approaches 100% reliability in determining fetal lung maturity
    b. lung surfactant phospholipids and approaches 80% reliability in determining fetal lung maturity
    c. fetal liver maturity by a spectrophotometric measurement
    d. brain cell development that has reached a level of maturity to sustain life outside the uterus

162   12. The L-S ratio greater than_____indicates maturity.
    a. 3:1   c. 2:1
    b. 4:1   d. 5:1

161   13. Genetic testing is recommended for all of the following reasons except
    a. the mother is over 35 years old
    b. there is a family history of genetic abnormalities
    c. to determine the sex of the child
    d. parents already have a child with a genetic abnormality

162 14. Meconium in amniotic fluid with amniocentesis indicates
   a. the fetus is in breech position
   b. the fetus may not getting enough oxygen
   c. the fetus has an abnormality in the gastrointestinal tract
   d. a normal finding

163 15. The amniotic fluid creatinine measures
   a. lung maturity
   b. liver maturity
   c. muscle mass and renal functioning
   d. anemia in the fetus

163 16. The biggest advantage of CVS is that
   a. it is a very accurate and complete chromosome study
   b. it is a very safe procedure with less risk than amniocentesis
   c. the procedure is performed early in the first trimester
   d. it is an easier test to perform than amniocentesis

160 17. AFP levels cannot be obtained through
   a. amniocentesis   c. serum blood samples at 16 weeks' gestation
   b. chorionic villi sampling d. serum blood samples at 18 weeks' gestation

FILL IN THE BLANK
Complete the following statements.

164 1. Ultrasound employ the use of _high freq._____ to obtain a visual
   picture of the fetus. _inaudible sounds_

166 2. Twenty-four hour urine estrogens are collected to evaluate _how well_
   placental function

167 3. A nonstress test is reactive if 2 or more fetal heart accelerations occur in a
   10- to 20-minute period. These accelerations should be greater than an increase of
   ___15___ beats per minute and last for _15_____

   _p166_ seconds or more.

SHORT ANSWERS

162–163 1. Name four tests that can be performed on amniotic fluid, and state what each test indicates.

a. _Meconium_ _____ _fetal distress_
   Degree of O2 recieving

b. _Lecithin-Sphingomyelin (L-S) Ratio_
   Lung surfactant phospholipids 100%

c. _Shake test_ _____ _rapid surfactant_
   test (done in 10 min)

d. _Amniotic fluid Creatinine—_
   muscle mass & renal function

163 2. What is the advantage of chorionic villi sampling over amniocentesis?

Done sooner

164 3. What is the main disadvantage of chorionic villi sampling compared with amniocentesis?

- AFP can't be taken

- ↑ risk of spontaneous abortion

- Not as complete & reliable

167–168   4. Explain "kick counts." Include how and when to count and what a positive or negative result might indicate.

10 – in 2 h period

MATCHING

1. Match the following tests with their descriptions.

163	2	a. CVS	1.	sample of fluid surrounding the fetus for chromosomal assessment
164	6	b. ultrasound	2.	cells taken from placental tissue
166–167	5	c. NST	3.	serum screen for neural tube defects
166	4	d. fetal blood sample	4.	sampling of blood from the fetus during labor
160	3	e. AFP	5.	a test based on the FHT and uterine contractions to determine fetal well-being
160–161	1	f. amniocentesis	6.	the use of sound waves to visualize the fetus

2. Match the desired information to the test used to obtain it. There may be more than one answer.

160   ___*1*___a. neural tube defect   1.   AFP

160   ___*3*___b. Down syndrome   2.   amniocentesis

161   _____c. lung maturity *2*   3.   triple screen

161   ___*2*___d. genetic abnormalities   4.   ultrasound

160 –166   _____e. structural abnormalities *4*

161–165   ___*4*___f. dating of fetus   *1 – CVS*

CASE STUDIES

1. Janice calls the office in her 37th week of pregnancy. She tells the nurse the baby has not been as active recently. What questions should the nurse ask Janice? What follow-up might be indicated and why?

2. Mary is a 38-year-old woman having an amniocentesis for genetic counseling. Describe to Mary in detail what she might expect from the procedure.

CHAPTER

10

The Stages and Mechanism of Labor and Delivery

MULTIPLE CHOICE
Select the one best answer.

cervix

stim hormone

oxytocin in

turn stim

more cont.

180   1. The cause of discomfort during labor is due to all the following except
   a. pull exerted on the cervix
   b. reduction of oxygen to muscles and tissue
   c. the pull of the ligaments with each contraction
   d. contraction of the uterine muscle

182   2. The sensation most commonly felt when a baby is in a posterior position is
   a. lower abdominal pull
   b. leg cramps
   c. back pain
   d. urge to push before full dilatation

182   3. The baby's head is delivered during
   a. extension   c. flexion
   b. external rotation   d. expulsion

184   4. Restitution occurs during
   a. expulsion   c. extension
   b. internal rotation   d. external rotation

178   5. The sacrum is designated by the letter(s)
   a. S   c. Sc
   b. M   d. Sa

179   6. If the baby's head is floating, it is said to be at _____ station.
   a. +4, +5   c. -3
   b. +3   d. -4,-5

179   7. The first stage of labor in the average primipara lasts
   a. 16 hours   c. 20 hours
   b. 24 hours   d. 12 hours

179   8. The time it takes for the cervix to dilate may depend on all of the following except
   a. age of the woman
   b. general health status of the woman
   c. number of previous pregnancies
   d. the amount of sleep the woman had before the onset of labor

176   9. The fourth stage of labor is known as the
   a. period of dilatation and effacement
   b. recovery stage
   c. placental stage
   d. period of expulsion

176–177 10. The most common attitude for a fetus to assume before labor is
   a. flexion   c. cephalic
   b. longitudinal   d. anterior

177–178 11. The most common lie for a fetus to assume before labor is
   a. flexion   c. cephalic
   b. longitudinal   d. anterior

178   12. The most common presentation for a fetus before labor is
   a. flexion   c. cephalic
   b. longitudinal   d. anterior

179   13. The most desirable position for birth is
   a. L.O.A.   c. R.O.T.
   b. L.O.P.   d. R.O.P.

173   14. When engagement takes place, all of the following occur except
   a. breathing becomes easier
   b. the fetus moves less
   c. walking and moving become more awkward
   d. urination becomes more frequent

174   15. Signs of early labor include all of the following except
        a.   show
        b.   rupture of membranes
        c.   light bleeding
        d.   regular contractions

175   16. The average contraction lasts
        a.   45–90 seconds   c.   30–45 seconds
        b.   1–2 minutes   d.   15–30 seconds

175   17. The peak of a contraction is called the
        a.   increment   c.   transition
        b.   decrement   d.   acme

176   18. All of the following suggest false labor except
        a.   irregular contractions
        b.   effacement and dilation
        c.   altered contraction pattern with a change of activity
        d.   contraction felt primarily in the lower abdomen

176   19. A completely dilated cervix is measured at
        a.   5 cm   c.   10 cm
        b.   8 cm   d.   12 cm

181   20. The second stage of labor begins when the
        a.   cervix is dilated 5–7 cm
        b.   cervix is dilated 8–10 cm
        c.   cervix is completely dilated
        d.   baby is born, and the placenta is being delivered

184   21. All of the following statements about an episiotomy are true except:
        a.   It substitutes a straight clean incision for a tear.
        b.   It shortens the duration of the second stage of labor.
        c.   It is necessary to avoid perineal tearing.
        d.   It spares the baby's head from pressure.

185   22. Immediately after the delivery of the placenta, the fundus can be located
        a.   halfway between the symphysis and the umbilicus
        b.   at the level of the umbilicus
        c.   just above the symphysis
        d.   halfway between the xiphoid and the umbilicus

173 23. When the presenting part of the fetus drops into the pelvis, it can be referred to as all of the following except

    a. lightening   c. 0 station

    b. engagement   d. quickening

175 24. The frequency of contractions are timed

    a. from the end of one contraction to the beginning of the next contraction

    b. from the beginning of one contraction to the beginning of the next contraction

    c. from the end of one contraction to the end of the next contraction

    d. from the beginning of one contraction to the end of the same contraction

176 25. The shortening of the cervical canal is called

    a. dilatation   c. true labor

    b. lightening   d. effacement

FILL IN THE BLANK

Complete the following statements.

174 1. The cervical mucous plug that is frequently streaked with blood is called ___Show___.

176 2. Effacement is measured in ___%___ ; dilatation is measured in ___cm___.

176 3. ___Effacement & Dilatation___ distinguishes true labor from false labor.

176 4. The first stage of labor begins with ___effacement___ and ends with ___dilation – complete.___

176 5. The second stage of labor begins with ___complete dilation___ and ends with ___delivery of fetus___.

176 6. The third stage of labor begins with ___birth___ and ends with ___expelled placenta + membrane.___

176 7. The fourth stage of labor begins with ___after birth of placenta___ and ends with ___last couple h after delivery.___

179 8. The degree of engagement of the presenting part of the fetus is called ___stations___.

181 9. The pressure of the baby's head against the cervix stimulates the release of the hormone ___oxytocin___, which in turn stimulates further contractions.

184 10. The incision of the perineum to facilitate delivery is called _episiotomy_.

184 11. After the baby's head is delivered, it rotates back 45 to 90 degrees, or until it resumes its normal relationship with the shoulders. This step is called _external_. _rotation restitution_

SHORT ANSWER

185 1. Why is it important to massage the uterus so that it remains hard after delivery?
hemorrhage

175 2. State the three stages of a uterine contraction.
   a. _Effacement & dilation_   _Phases_
   b. _Expulsion_   _increment_
   c. _Placenta_   _acme_
                    decrement

173 3. Name three possible signs that labor is about to begin.
   a. _Show_   _lightening_
   b. _ROM_
   c. _Contractions – regular_

181 4. The first stage of labor is divided into three phases. Name each phase and the degree of dilatation in each.
   a. _Latent_   _1 – 4_ cm
   b. _accelerated_   _5 – 7_ cm
   c. _transition_   _8 – 10_ cm

185 5. Name six things the nurse should check during the fourth stage of labor.
   a. _Lochia_   d. _VS_
   b. _Urine_   e. _flow of blood_
   c. _fundus_   f. _bladder empty completely_

MATCHING

182 1. List in order the mechanism of labor.
   a. _4_   1. internal rotation   _restitution_
   b. _6_   2. external rotation
   c. _2_   3. descent
   d. _3_   4. flexion
   e. _7_   5. expulsion
   f. _5_   6. extension
   g. _1_   7. engagement

2. Match the terms in the left column with their definitions in the right column.

177   ___2___   a. lie   1. the relationship of the fetus body to itself

178   ___4___   b. position   2. the relationship of the long axis of the fetus to that of the mother

176–177   ___1___   c. attitude   3. the part of the fetus that enters the internal cervical os for delivery

178   ___3___   d. presentation   4. the part of the fetus to the right or left of the mother

LABELING

Label the categories of presentations in the following illustration.

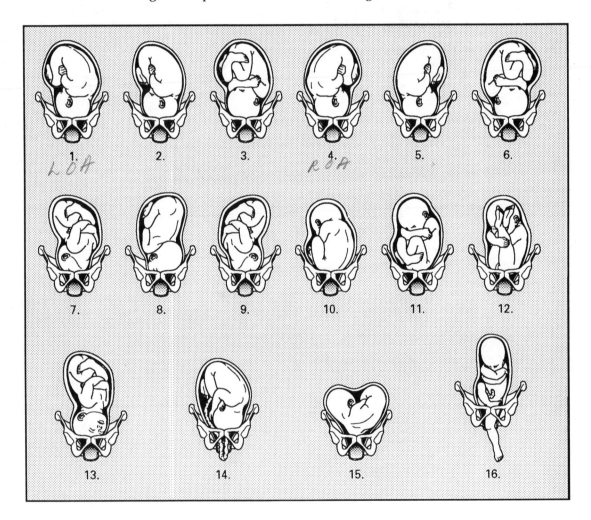

1. LOA   2.   3.   4. ROA   5.   6.

7.   8.   9.   10.   11.   12.

13.   14.   15.   16.

1. _____   9. _____

2. _____   10. _____

3. _____   11. _____

4. _____   12. _____

5. _____   13. _____

6. _____   14. _____

7. _____   15. _____

8. _____   16. _____

EXERCISES

1. Practice determining the fetal position by using the Leopold's maneuvers.
2. Practice measuring fetal growth by using a tape measure from the pubic symphysis to the top of the uterus (fundus).

CASE STUDY

174   Joyce is a 25-year-old primigravida who calls her physician's office at 39.5 weeks' gestation. She reports waking up in a puddle of fluid. As the nurse screening the call, what questions would you ask Joyce? What advice would you give her and why?

CHAPTER

11

Management of the Patient in Labor

MULTIPLE CHOICE
Select the one best answer.

196   1. An enema is sometimes given during early labor for all of the following reasons except to
   a. relieve constipation
   b. empty the rectum and reduce obstruction of baby's movement
   c. reduce abdominal cramping
   d. stimulate uterine contractions

200   2. All of the following affect the rapidity of labor and delivery except the
   a. size and position of the baby
   b. mother's pelvic measurement
   c. rupture of membranes
   d. health of the fetus

190   3. All of the following information is needed upon admission of a laboring woman except the
   a. pattern of labor
   b. state of bag of waters
   c. last bowel movement
   d. expected date of confinement

192   4. Blood pressure is usually taken every _____ during labor.
   a. hour   c. 2 hours
   b. 15 minutes   d. 4 hours

192   5. All of the following information about uterine contractions should be reported except

      a. frequency   c. duration

      b. intensity   d. fetal movement during a contraction

192   6. A contraction that could lead to fetal hypoxia lasts longer than _____ seconds.

      a. 60   c. 45

      b. 90   d. 30

192–193   7. Abdominal palpation is performed to check all of the following except the

      a. position   c. size of baby

      b. presentation   d. station

193   8. FHT are checked by using any of the following except

      a. fetoscope   c. doppler

      b. stethoscope   d. electron fetal monitor

200   9. The definition of a prolapsed cord can include all of the following except one that

      a. lies beside the presenting part at the pelvic inlet

      b. descends into the vagina

      c. passes out of the vagina

      d. the fetus compresses

200   10. The simplest effective method of inducing labor is

      a. nipple stimulation   c. pitocin

      b. enema   d. amniotomy

201   11. The function of prostaglandin is to

      a. lower blood pressure

      b. soften the cervix

      c. delay labor

      d. reduce pain

201   12. The function of an oxytocin drug is to

      a. lower blood pressure

      b. soften the cervix

      c. induce contractions

      d. reduce pain

192   13. If a laboring woman's pulse is over 100 beats per minute, the nurse should

      a. check for an overly distended bladder

      b. suspect dehydration

      c. assume this is normal with pain

      d. suspect PIH

FILL IN THE BLANK

Complete the following statements.

194   1. The fetal heart rate normally ranges from _120_ to _160_ beats per minute.

204   2. The purpose of IV fluids during labor is _forstall dehydration & exhaustion_.

193–194 3. During a contraction, the FHT will normally _↓_ but return to normal rate after the contraction ends.

196   4. The major disadvantage of shaving the perineal area may be the risk of _infection_.

200   5. A prolapsed cord is more commonly found with babies in _breech_ position.

200   6. The position the woman should assume if the cord is found to be prolapsed is _Knee-chest or side_.

SHORT ANSWER

190   1. Name five things the nurse should ask the laboring woman upon admission to the hospital.
    a. _ROM_
    b. _EDC_
    c. _Show_
    d. _Time & freq. of contractions_
    e. _# of preg. & any previous comp._

191–194 2. Name four things the nurse should physically check upon admitting the laboring woman to the hospital.
    a. _Durat., freq, intensity_
    b. _Show_
    c. _Urine_
    d. _VS_

191–194 3. Name six abnormal findings indicating labor is not progressing normally.
    a. _bleeding_
    b. _late decceleration_
    c. _prolong. contraction_

d. *↑ or ↓ of FHT*

e. *prolapsed cord*

f. *↑ UVS of mother   PIH*

200   4. Name four reasons why a physician might elect to induce labor.

a. *PID*

b. *diabetes*

c. *hydramnios*

d. *fetal distress*

200   5. List two common methods of inducing labor.

a. *ROM*   b. *Pitocin*

amniocent

201   6. Describe three things the nurse can do to make the patient more comfortable in the first stage of labor.

a. *Explain & encourage*

b. *CKUS*

c. *Coach*

191   7. In a chart, after TPAL, appear the numbers 2–0–1–2. What does this mean?

T 2 terms

0 prem

1 abortion

2 living

196   8. List three reasons why perineal preparation might be done.

a. *episiotomy easier*

b. *ensure quicker healing & cleanliness*

c. *prevent infection*

Better view

198–199 9. List one advantage and one disadvantage of each of the following positions used during labor.

a. Standing   Advantage: _____

               Disadvantage: _____

b. Walking   Advantage: _____

               Disadvantage: _____

c. Semisitting   Advantage: _____

Disadvantage: _____

d. Sitting upright   Advantage: _____

Disadvantage: _____

e. Hands and knees   Advantage: _____

Disadvantage: _____

f. Side-lying   Advantage: _____

Disadvantage: _____

g. Squatting   Advantage: _____

Disadvantage: _____

h. Back-lying   Advantage: _____

Disadvantage: _____

200   10. What is the major risk of a prolapsed cord?

Lack of blood flow

ACTIVITIES

194   1. Describe the rectal exam procedure and what is being evaluated.

_____

_____

195   2. Describe the vaginal exam procedure and what is being evaluated.

_____

_____

197   3. Describe the catheterization procedure.

_____

_____

CASE STUDY

Mary has been admitted to the hospital in labor and is found to be dilated to 7 cm. Her husband is her support coach, and Mary and her husband attended childbirth preparation classes. They are trying to have their baby without medication or intervention. Her labor is progressing normally without complications. Create a nursing care plan for Mary, addressing at least five different issues.

Fetal Monitoring

MULTIPLE CHOICE
Select the one best answer.

209
1. If the FHT is listened to with a fetal stethoscope every 15 minutes for a duration of 30 seconds, approximately ___ percent of information is obtained.
   a. 30
   b. 60
   c. 3
   d. 15

210
2. The most common cause of fetal distress is/are
   a. placenta abruptio
   b. sustained uterine contractions
   c. umbilical cord compression
   d. maternal medications

211
3. The phonotransducer measures
   a. uterine contractions
   b. fetal movements
   c. fetal heart tones
   d. intensity of contractions

215
4. Minimal variability of the fetal heart rate at the baseline may indicate all of the following except
   a. nervous system hypoxia
   b. prematurity
   c. presence of drugs in the fetal circulation
   d. autonomic control

223
5. The purpose of fetal blood sampling is to
   a. test for fetal maturity
   b. test for fetal distress
   c. test oxygen blood levels
   d. test for Rh antibodies

209 6. The earliest references to fetal observation for distress can be found in literature as early as the

    a. 1600s   c. 1800s

    b. 1700s   d. early 1900s

209 7. The first successful recording of fetal ECG through the mother's abdomen was reported by Hon in

    a. 1891   c. 1957

    b. 1908   d. 1964

210 8. Fetal monitoring during labor gives all the following information except

    a. early detection of fetal distress

    b. early detection of abnormal uterine contractions

    c. predicting the length of labor

    d. detecting umbilical cord compression

210–211 9. The indirect method of monitoring includes all of the following except

    a. uterine activity transducer   c. phonotransducer

    b. ECG electrode   d. Doppler transducer

211 10. The uterine activity transducer responds to

    a. fetal movements

    b. fetal heart movements

    c. muscle tone in the abdominal wall

    d. cervical dilatation

213 11. Between the 8th and 11th week of pregnancy, the average fetal pulse rate is

    a. 120–160 beats per minute   c. 170–179 beats per minute

    b. 100–120 beats per minute   d. 140–158 beats per minute

FILL IN THE BLANK

Complete the following statements.

210 1. Fetal monitoring is accomplished by either _direct_ methods or _indirect_ methods.

211 2. External geometrical changes may be detected by a transducer called a _tocotransducer_ strapped to the patient's abdomen.

212 3. A transducer that detects fetal heart movement and is insensitive to other maternal noises is called a _doppler_ .

214-215 4. The top half of the monitor screen represents _F H R_ ; the bottom half tracts _contraction increment - acme - decrement_

216 5. The variability of the fetal heart rate baseline reflects _automatic control_ .

215 6. A heart rate of less than 120 beats per minute is called fetal _bradycardia_.

215 7. A heart rate of more than 160 beats per minute is called fetal _tachycardia_.

218 8. Late decelerations are a probable indication of _fetal distress_ _uteroplacental insufficiency_

220 9. If late decelerations develop during the oxytocin challenge test, the test is called _+_ and suggests diminished _uteroplacental reserve_ .

SHORT ANSWER

213 1. Name four indications for which the Doppler transducer has been found to be helpful.
   a. _Early detection of pregnancy_
   b. _Diagnosis of fetal death in utero_
   c. _Detection of a remote fetal heartbeat_
   d. _Intermittent observation of the rate & rhythm of fetal pulse_

213 2. List four conditions with which direct monitoring cannot be used.
   a. _Placenta previa_
   b. _Premature labor_
   c. _Second twins_
   d. _Unruptured membrane_

214 3. Name three conditions that can be detected by fetal heart pattern readings.
   a. _____
   b. _____
   c. _____

215   4. Name four conditions that may be responsible for fetal tachycardia.

       a. *Immaturity*

       b. *maternal fever*

       c. *Minimal fetal hypoxia*

       d. *fetal distress*

215   5. Describe what the fetal monitor will reveal about uterine contractions.

      Increment, acme, decrement
      baseline tone, freq, duration intensity

216   6. Define acute fetal distress.

    1. Late decelerations of any severity

    2. Variable decelerations that last more than 1 min, — fetal HR ↓ to 60 b.p.m. or less
    Fetal compromise related to the recurring stress of uterine contractions n umbilical cord compression

219   7. If the nurse sees variable decelerations, what can the nurse do to see if this pattern can be alleviated?

    Change Mom's position Monitor VS & FHR Administer O₂

218   8. If the nurse sees late decelerations, what might be ordered by the physician to compensate?

    O₂ or atropine

220   9. During the oxytocin challenge test, what contraction pattern is expected?

    3 contractions in 10 mins period

220   10. List four indications for performing an oxytocin challenge test. *28 wks*

       a. *Diabetes*

       b. *PIH*

       c. *preeclampsia*

       d. *Intrauterine growth retardation*

       Rh sensitized
       stillborn history

220   11. List three contraindications to the oxytocin challenge test.

      a. _Premature RM_

      b. _Placenta previa_

      c. _C/S Cesarean_

      Premature labor history

220   12. Explain the results of a reactive nonstress test.

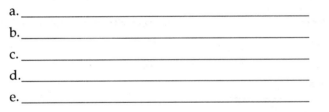

Reacts to fetal movement 15 bpm above baseline & lasts 15 sec.

220–223   13. Name two advantages of the NST over the OCT.

      a. _Economical_

      b. _Non invasive_

210   14. List five Category I conditions that require close and accurate fetal monitoring.

      a. _____

      b. _____

      c. _____

      d. _____

      e. _____

223   15. Briefly describe the placement of a direct fetal monitor and an intrauterine catheter.

223, 225–226 16. Name one advantage and one disadvantage of fetal blood sampling.

MATCHING
Match the condition with what is most likely to be indicated on the fetal monitor.

216   _2_ a. irregularity of baseline
fetal heart rate

                                          1. immaturity, maternal fever, and fetal hypoxia

215   _1_ b. fetal tachycardia   2. immaturity of autonomic nervous system

217   _4_ c. prolonged variable
deceleration   3. congenital heart lesions

217   _3_ d. pure bradycardia   4. fetal distress, cord compression

217   _5_ e. accelerations   5. may occur without fetal jeopardy

217–218   _6_ f. early decelerations   6. head compression

EXERCISE
Obtain a variety of fetal and uterine monitoring strips, and evaluate them in detail with the help of an experienced interpreter.

13 | *Pain Relief for Labor and Delivery*

MULTIPLE CHOICE
Select the one best answer.

234   1. A saddle block is similar to a
    a. caudal   c. spinal
    b. epidural   d. local

235   2. A pudendal block is administered during the
    a. first stage of labor
    b. second stage of labor
    c. third stage of labor
    d. third phase of the first stage of labor *transition*

234   3. An epidural block can cause a change in the mother's blood pressure. Preventive measures to avoid this include
    a. administering IV fluids
    b. positioning the mother in an upright or semi-sitting position
    c. decreasing the amount of medication given
    d. asking the woman to drink water throughout her labor

234   4. Spinal anesthesia is given during the
    a. first stage of labor
    b. second stage of labor
    c. third stage of labor
    d. second phase of the first stage of labor

234   5. Spinal anesthesia is used for all the following except
    a. cesarean section
    b. forceps delivery
    c. to relax the perineal floor in a difficult delivery

d. to repair an episiotomy

232   6. Caudal anesthesia was first applied to childbirth in
    a. 1909   c. 1927
    b. 1886   d. 1952

232   7. Regional anesthesia is usually not given to the primigravida until her cervix is dilated to
    a. >4 cm   c. >7 cm
    b. >6 cm   d. >8 cm

232   8. Which of the following can be given continuously as regional anesthesia?
    a. spinal   c. caudal
    b. paracervical   d. local

231   9. General anesthesia is commonly used
    a. during the first stage of labor
    b. only in situations that require rapid delivery
    c. because it doesn't adversely affect the fetus
    d. because it is easily administered by the obstetrician through the IV

231   10. Side effects attributable to regional anesthesia include
    a. nausea and vomiting   c. drop in blood pressure
    b. drowsiness   d. rapid heart beat

232   11. If a woman is given a caudal anesthesia, all of the following need to be carefully monitored except
    a. uterine contractions   c. bladder fullness
    b. fetal movements   d. blood pressure

230   12. An example of an injectable or oral medication prescribed to reduce anxiety and relax the woman is
    a. Sparine   c. Penthrane
    b. Scopolamine   d. Trilene

231   13. All of the following are true about narcotic analgesics except that they
    a. relieve pain
    b. sedate and reduce anxiety
    c. increase rate of cervical dilatation
    d. depress neonatal respirations

230   14. Medication labeling is required regarding all the following except
    a. effects on the mother's milk
    b. cited studies that prove side effects

c. likelihood of need for intervention during labor and delivery

d. effects on later growth and development

231 15. Analgesia is designed to

a. give total loss of sensation

b. bring about partial loss of sensation

c. completely stop pain

d. lessen pain perception

231 16. The following statements are true about anesthesia except that it

a. refers to total loss of sensation

b. may cause loss of consciousness

c. may block specific area from pain

d. does not affect the fetus

231 17. Administered during the second stage of labor, this medication affects the entire system and may be passed to the fetus.

a. regional anesthesia

b. general anesthesia

c. local anesthesia

d. systemic analgesia

231 18. General anesthesia is

a. administered by the obstetrician

b. administered by the nurse

c. administered by the anesthesiologist

d. self-administered

232 19. What must be monitored closely when anesthesia is administered?

a. baby's movements

b. progress of labor

c. blood pressure

d. mother's respirations

234 20. A spinal headache can be avoided by

a. having an anesthesiologist administer the medication

b. giving the woman IV fluids

c. having the woman remain flat in bed for 4–8 hours after delivery

d. using less medication

235 21. The most effective medication given for an episiotomy is

(a.) local anesthesia   c. paracervical
b. pudendal   d. caudal

FILL IN THE BLANK
Complete the following statements.

234 1. The anesthetic that can possibly cause a headache is
        Spinal & saddle.

230 2. Medications that offer relief of pain without loss of sensation is called
        Analgesia.

230 3. Medications that offer a loss of sensation or consciousness are called
        anesthesia.

SHORT ANSWER

241 1. List four characteristic signs of prelabor.
        a. _____
        b. _____
        c. _____
        d. _____

241 2. List seven signs of transition (third phase of the first stage of labor).
        a. _Strong Contractions_
        b. _Pressure on rectum_
        c. _Cramp_
        d. _Nausea_
        e. _Uncontrollable Shaking_
        f. _Irritability_
        g. _Urge to Push_

234 3. What causes a spinal headache?
        Leakage of fluid thru puncture in dura

235 4. Explain the fear-tension-pain syndrome.

233   5.   Name three advantages of the epidural over the caudal block.

       a. *Less medication needed*

       b. *takes effect sooner*

       c. *Less risk of infection*

230   6.   List four of the FDA's labeling requirements for medication used during labor and delivery.

       a. *Long + Short term effects*

       b. *Effect on duration of labor & delivery*

       c. *Intervention - forceps*

       d. *Effect on growth, development, mothers milk*

231   7.   Describe two situations that might occur in labor that would necessitate the need for general anesthesia.

       a. *fetal distress*

       b. *Intrauterine manipulation is required*

235–236   8.   Describe three things the nurse can do to help the laboring woman.

       a. *Encourage + relax*

       b. *Message back*

       c. *Cold / heat on/off*

MATCHING

1.   Match the following medications with their effects.

233	3	a. epidural	1.	loss of sensation of cervical dilation
234	4	b. spinal	2.	a numbing effect from waist down; administered in the lower spine
231	1	c. paracervical	3.	a numbing effect from waist down; administered in the lumbar region outside the dura sac
232	2	d. caudal	4.	medication used most often for a cesarean section
235	5	e. pudendal	5.	medication with numbing effect on the perineum and vagina

2. Match the following medications with their classification. More than one drug may be in the same class.

230   _1_   a. Vistaril   1. sedative

230   _2_   b. Seconal   2. barbiturate

231   _4_   c. Demerol   3. amnesic

230   _1_   d. Phenergan   4. narcotic

230   _3_   e. Scopolamine

CASE STUDY

Judy is a primigravida in labor with her cervix at 6 centimeters. She was just given a caudal anesthesia by the anesthesiologist. Design a nursing care plan for the remainder of Judy's labor. Consider both Judy and her baby in the care plan.

CHAPTER 14

Nursing Care in Delivery

MATCHING
Select the one best answer.

243   1. All of the following suggest the beginning of the second stage of labor except
    a.   intense contractions occurring rapidly and lasting 60–90 seconds
    b.   nausea
    c.   slowdown of contractions and a rest period
    d.   perspiration on the upper lip

243   2. During the desire to push, the nurse should instruct the mother to
    a.   take deep chest breaths
    b.   take short, even breaths
    c.   bear down with each contraction until crowning
    d.   hold her breath through the entire contraction

251   3. Forceps or the vacuum extractor may need to be used in all the following situations except
    a.   when FHT slows or becomes irregular
    b.   when the baby's position makes delivery difficult
    c.   to help in the delivery of a breech position
    d.   when the mother is too tired to push any longer

253   4. The need for an episiotomy is dependent upon
    a.   the physician's routine practice
    b.   the size of the baby
    c.   the elasticity of the perineal tissue
    d.   whether the mother is a primipara or a multipara

259   5. If the baby does not cry spontaneously immediately after birth, the doctor may
      a. hold the baby's head downward and rub its back
      b. hold the baby up by the heels so mucous drains and gently tap the baby's back
      c. resuscitate the baby with the available equipment
      d. wait for 60–90 seconds for the baby to breathe on its own before doing anything

256   6. Leboyer births include all of the following except
      a. no unnecessary stimulation
      b. little handling of the newborn
      c. soft lights
      d. gentle, controlled delivery

257   7. Immediately after birth, the nurse should
      a. place the baby in a heated incubator
      b. take the baby to the head of the table for the mother to see and hold
      c. note the exact time of delivery
      d. suction the baby

258   8. An absence of the Moro reflex is a possible result of
      a. intracranial pathology   c. hypoglycemia
      b. prematurity   d. Down syndrome

258   9. If the baby's nails, umbilical cord, and vernix appear yellow stained, this suggests
      a. anemia   c. previous fetal distress
      b. blood incompatibility   d. viral infection

258   10. A diaphragmatic hernia will be suspected if
      a. little or no Moro reflex is observed
      b. bowel sounds are heard in the chest
      c. the heart rate is >160 beats per minute
      d. no meconium is expelled after birth

259   11. Antibiotic or 1% silver nitrate is put into the newborn's eyes to
      a. protect the infant's eyes from infectious organisms that may have been in the birth canal
      b. help the newborn focus better
      c. protect the infant's eyes from infectious organisms that he or she may be exposed to after birth
      d. treat an existing infection

259   12. The Apgar score is given to the newborn
- a. immediately after birth and again at 10 minutes
- b. within the first minute after birth
- c. at 1 minute and at 5 minutes after birth
- d. at 5 minutes and at 10 minutes after birth

259   13. The most important responsibility of the obstetrical nurse after a delivery is to observe the newborn closely for
- a. irritability
- b. listlessness
- c. respiratory or circulatory depression
- d. congenital deformities

261   14. Blood loss is considered a hemorrhage if it exceeds
- a. 200 mL
- b. 300 mL
- c. 400 mL
- d. 500 mL

262   15. If the baby is put on the mother's abdomen immediately after delivery, this will help accomplish all of the following except
- a. skin-to-skin contact supplying warmth to the baby
- b. facilitating bonding
- c. helping the uterus stay firm
- d. facilitating mucus drainage from the baby

261   16. Oxytocin administered intramuscularly after delivery
- a. reduces pain
- b. increases uterine contractions
- c. prevents milk production if the mother chooses not to nurse her baby
- d. produces a sedative effect

261   17. To relieve discomfort and swelling of an episiotomy, the nurse should
- a. apply heat to the area
- b. offer medication
- c. apply pressure with a sanitary pad
- d. apply ice to the area

256   18. The childbirth method that encourages a gentle, controlled delivery and avoidance of overstimulation of the newborn is called
- a. Lamaze
- b. Bradley
- c. Leboyer
- d. Lawrence

FILL IN THE BLANK
Complete the following statements.

261 1. Nursing care during the third stage of labor includes recording the exact time the
placenta is delivered; observing the mother for
hemorrhage and _shock_ ; observing the baby for
Breathing _mucus_, _color_, and
cry.

261 2. The placenta is processed for the recovery and purification of
gamma _globulin_, a serum used in the prevention
and treatment of a variety of diseases.

243 3. When the largest diameter of the baby's head is in the vaginal opening, it is called
crowning.

259 4. The earliest evaluation of extrauterine life of the newborn is scored and is called the
Apgar score. A perfect score totals _10_.

SHORT ANSWER

246 1. Two key concepts help guide a mother and her support team through the second
stage of labor. They are:
a. _Not pushing_
b. _Follow body signals_

247–251 2. Name one advantage and one disadvantage for each of the following positions used
in the second stage of labor.

a. Semisitting   Advantage: _____

Disadvantage: _____

b. Side-lying   Advantage: _____

Disadvantage: _____

c. Lying on back   Advantage: _____

Disadvantage: _____

d. Squatting   Advantage: _____

Disadvantage: _____

e. Supported squat   Advantage: _____

Disadvantage: _____

f. Semi-lithotomy   Advantage: _____

Disadvantage: _____

g. Lithotomy   Advantage: _____

Disadvantage: _____

253   3. Define bonding and how it occurs.

253   4. Explain in detail how to instruct a woman in the second stage of labor to most effectively push her baby out.

255   5. Name three differences between delivering in a standard hospital room and in an alternative birthing center.

        a. _____

        b. _____

        c. _____

256   6. List three goals of the newborn examination.

        a. _____

        b. _____

        c. _____

256   7. List six areas to be closely evaluated in the newborn assessment.

        a. _____   d. _____

        b. _____   e. _____

        c. _____   f. _____

262   8. Name five signs that should be closely monitored in the mother during the fourth
          stage of labor.

          a. _____

          b. _____

          c. _____

          d. _____

          e. _____

263   9. List four things that are assessed daily during the postpartum hospital stay for the
          mother and for the baby.

          Mother   Baby

          a. _____   _____

          b. _____   _____

          c. _____   _____

          d. _____   _____

243   10. List six indications in the laboring woman that suggest the second stage of labor is
          beginning.

          a. _____

          b. _____

          c. _____

          d. _____

          e. _____

          f. _____

243   11. Whether a woman delivers in a birthing room or in a delivery room, list the
          equipment the nurse should have set up.

          a. _____   f. _____

          b. _____   g. _____

          c. _____   h. _____

          d. _____   i. _____

          e. _____

246   12. What two factors make the pushing efforts by the mother most effective?

          a. _____

          b. _____

251   13. The physician can help the delivery process with a choice of what two instruments?

        a. _____   b. _____

251–252 14. Explain three reasons for an episiotomy.

        a. _____

        b. _____

        c. _____

259   15. Name three observations suggesting respiratory distress in the newborn.

        a. _____

        b. _____

        c. _____

259   16. What is the purpose of infant eye treatment following delivery?

        _____

260   17. Name the five areas evaluated in the Apgar scoring system.

        a. _____

        b. _____

        c. _____

        d. _____

        e. _____

263–264 18. Name three topics that should be addressed with the new parents upon discharge from the hospital.

        a. _____

        b. _____

        c. _____

EXERCISE

Research and write a short paper about a newborn's ability to interact and respond to various stimuli. Discuss how bonding attachment occurs.

CASE STUDY

Susie is a 22-year-old woman who has just delivered a 7-pound, 6-ounce baby boy. This is her first child and she and her husband are elated. Write a nursing care plan for Susie during her fourth stage of labor. Write a nursing care plan for Susie's baby during the fourth stage of labor. What issues need to be addressed with Susie and her husband before discharge from the hospital?

CHAPTER 15

Complications of Labor and Delivery

MULTIPLE CHOICE

Select the one best answer.

267   1. A labor is termed premature if it begins _____ or more weeks before the expected date.
    a. 3   c. 4
    b. 2   d. 6

267   2. Lung maturity can be diagnosed by
    a. amniocentesis to determine L-S ratio
    b. ultrasound
    c. fetal blood sampling
    d. biophysical profile

267–268   3. To induce the baby's lungs to mature, _____ can be given.
    a. oxytocin   c. antibiotics
    b. steroids   d. tocolytics

268   4. The cause of PROM (premature rupture of membranes) includes all of the following except
    a. trauma (coitus or pelvic exam)
    b. incompetent cervix
    c. polyhydramnios
    d. amniotomy

268   5. The management of choice in PROM in close-to-term pregnancies is
    a. cesarean section
    b. wait and watch approach
    c. induction
    d. forceps delivery

269   6. Dystocia is defined as
    a. fast delivery   c. slow labor
    b. difficult labor   d. complicated delivery

269   7. Uterine dystocia can be managed in all of the following ways except
    a. sedate the mother to allow her to rest
    b. stimulate contractions
    c. eliminate the risk of dehydration
    d. allow the labor to progress without intervention of any kind

271–272   8. Brow or face presentations are diagnosed by all of the following techniques except
    a. pelvic exam
    b. ultrasound
    c. meconium stained amniotic fluid
    d. roentgenography

269   9. Minor degrees of pelvic contractions can be overcome by all of the following except
    a. efficient uterine contractions
    b. expansion of soft tissue
    c. favorable birth position
    d. breaking the bag of waters

274   10. Approximately _____ percent of hospital deliveries in the United States are cesarean sections.
    a. 6   c. >30
    b. 10–20   d. 2

276   11. Prerequisites for a safe VBAC include all of the following except
    a. parents' informed consent
    b. no indications recommending a repeat cesarean
    c. labor is induced so it can be controlled
    d. backup facilities for immediate cesarean section are available

278   12. Prolapsed cord is a complication that occurs in
    a. 1:200 births   c. 1:1,000 births
    b. 1:400 births   d. 1:2,000 births

278   13. If the nurse discovers a prolapsed cord, she should do all of the following except
    a. put the mother in Trendelenburg or knee-chest position
    b. apply pressure against the presenting part away from the cord
    c. try to gently replace the cord back into the uterus
    d. notify the physician immediately

278   14. If bleeding is present during labor, a placenta previa may be suspected. Determining a placenta previa can be accomplished by
- a. ultrasound
- b. pelvic exam
- c. waiting for the placenta to be delivered first
- d. x-ray

280   15. Bleeding is concealed in placenta abruptio in _____ percent of cases.
- a. 20
- b. 30
- c. 5
- d. 10

281   16. In a normal vaginal delivery, there is an expected blood loss of approximately
- a. 500 mL
- b. 200–300 mL
- c. 50–100 mL
- d. 750 mL

281–282   17. Indications that postpartum hemorrhage is occurring include all of the following signs except
- a. rapid weak pulse
- b. shortness of breath
- c. fever
- d. falling blood pressure

283–284   18. When caring for the newly delivered unconscious mother, all of the following are checked and recorded except
- a. rate and character of respirations
- b. color and condition of skin
- c. blood pressure
- d. temperature

267   19. Which of the following has the greatest effect on premature survival?
- a. gestational age
- b. weight
- c. intrauterine stress
- d. age of the mother

267   20. Usually lung maturity is adequate for survival by
- a. 27 weeks
- b. 38 weeks
- c. 32 weeks
- d. 35 weeks

268   21. Premature rupture of membranes is defined as
        a. spontaneous rupture one hour or more prior to the onset of labor
        b. spontaneous rupture before 38 weeks' gestation
        c. rupture of the membranes before the fetus is mature enough for extrauterine life
        d. spontaneous rupture of the membranes when the fetal birth weight would indicate prematurity

269   22. A precipitous labor is defined as one that lasts
        a. less than 1 hour   c. less than 3 hours
        b. less than 6 hours   d. more than 30 hours

269–270 23. A persistent occiput posterior position is suspected if the mother has
        a. prolonged labor
        b. ineffective contractions
        c. back pain
        d. meconium-stained amniotic fluid

280   24. Severe abruptio of the placenta is categorized by
        a. <100 mL blood loss; uterine activity increased slightly; no change in FHT
        b. bleeding 100–500 mL; uterine tone increased; FHT suggests distress
        c. bleeding 100–500 mL; uterus is hypersensitive; FHT indicates distress
        d. bleeding >500 mL; uterus tetanic; fetal distress evident

270–271 25. The most common medical management for breech-positioned babies is
        a. turn the baby during labor (version)
        b. deliver the baby in breech position vaginally
        c. perform a cesarean section
        d. perform a large episiotomy for extra room

FILL IN THE BLANK
Complete the following statements.

268   1. The nitrazine test is one of the easiest ways to determine
        _____PROM_____.

268   2. Amniotic fluid is _____alkaline_____ (pH) than vaginal or cervical secretions.

269   3. A delay in any of the phases of labor is known as _____uterine dysfunction_____.

278 4. The cord coiled around the baby's neck at the time of delivery is called _nuchal cord_.

267 5. The most common cause of morbidity and mortality in premature infants is _Lung immaturity_

275 6. The preferred incision for a cesarean section is _Transverse incision_.

SHORT ANSWER

268 1. If a baby is born prematurely, special attention needs to be focused in what four basic areas?
   a. _Warm/dry_
   b. _Handle to care_
   c. _Protected from infection_
   d. _Helped to breathe_

268 2. Explain the fern test in evaluating amniotic fluid.

Amniotic fluid shows up in a fern pattern when dried

269 3. Explain the difference between precipitous labor and precipitous delivery.

Sudden labor <3 h. Delivery sudden + unexpected + sometimes un attended.

270 4. To lessen back pain in a persistent occiput-positioned labor, the nurse should
   a. _Change position_
   b. _message back._

273–274　5. Briefly describe the usual medical management of a multiple gestation delivery if

　　　a.　the first baby is in breech position: _____

　　　　　_____

　　　b.　the labor begins before the 32nd week gestation:_____

　　　　　_____

　　　　　_____

　　　c.　the first baby is in vertex position: _____

　　　　　_____

　　　d.　there are three or more babies:_____

　　　　　_____

267　6. List three interventions to attempt to arrest premature labor.

　　　a._____

　　　b._____

　　　c._____

268　7. Name two risks of premature rupture of membranes.

　　　a._____

　　　b._____

269　8. Name five possible reasons for a precipitous labor.

　　　a._____

　　　b._____

　　　c._____

　　　d._____

　　　e._____

269　9. List three possible reasons for a prolonged labor.

　　　a._____

　　　b._____

　　　c._____

272　10. The usual medical management of labor with a brow presentation is _____

　　　_____

273　11. Define fetopelvic disproportion.

　　　_____

273   12. Name five conditions for which a woman is at higher risk when she has a multiple pregnancy.

      a. _____   d. _____

      b. _____   e. _____

      c. _____

275   13. Briefly explain why a transverse lower uterine segment incision (suprasymphyeal incision) is preferred when doing a cesarean section.

276   14. The letters VBAC are defined as

      a.   V: _*Vaginal*_____

      b.   B: _*Birth*_____

      c.   A: _*After*_____

      d.   C: _*Cesarean*_____

278   15. Name three conditions that may make a prolapsed cord more likely to occur.

      a. _____

      b. _____

      c. _____

280   16. List three symptoms the woman may exhibit if she has a placenta abruptio.

      a. _*Bleeding*_____

      b. _*Pain in uterus & lower back*_____

      c. _*Uterine hypertonicity*_____

281   17. Define postpartum hemorrhage.

281   18. Name three signs or symptoms that may indicate postpartum hemorrhage.

    a._____

    b._____

    c._____

282   19. Name four possible causes of postpartum hemorrhage.

    a._____

    b._____

    c._____

    d._____

282   20. Anoxia is a common cause of stillbirth. Name four conditions that may create anoxia for the fetus.

    a._____

    b._____

    c._____

    d._____

MATCHING

270   Match the following breech positions to the correct definitions.

_____ a. footling   1. buttocks and feet present with knees drawn up

_____ b. frank   2. one or both feet present

_____ c. complete   3. legs extended up and pressed against abdomen and chest

CASE STUDIES

1. Judy has been in active labor for 22 hours. Her cervix is dilated to 6 cm and is 100% effaced. Her contractions remain regular at 1 to 2 minutes apart. She remains unmedicated. She has made no progress in the past four hours. What are the possible reasons for Judy's long labor? What is the possible medical management of this labor? What can the nurse do to make Judy more comfortable?

2. The patient you are caring for is scheduled for an unexpected Cesarean section. Describe how you would explain the procedure to her. What would you tell her about medication, recovery, and breast feeding?

Postpartum Care

MULTIPLE CHOICE
Select the one best answer.

289   1. The most significant sign in determining the importance of a low grade fever during the fourth stage of labor is

     a.   blood pressure   c.   urine output

     b.   respirations   d.   pulse

291   2. The usual period of time for involution to be complete is

     a. 3 weeks   c. 6 weeks

     b. 4 weeks   d. 8 weeks

290   3. The normal flow of vaginal blood within the first two hours after delivery is approximately

     a.   2 oz   c.   3 oz

     b.   <1 oz   d.   >5 oz

290   4. It is not uncommon for a newly delivered woman to experience a chill after labor. This chill usually is caused by

     a.   the cold environment of the delivery room

     b.   a slowed heart rate after delivery

     c.   a disturbance of internal and external temperature due to excessive perspiration during labor

     d.   excitement of having just delivered a baby

298   5. Psychological manifestations such as personality changes and postpartum depression can occur when a woman

     a.   is deprived of sleep

     b.   has had a particularly long and difficult labor

     c.   has gone a long period of time without food during her labor

     d.   has had large amounts of various medications during her labor

281   6. A woman who has had a cesarean birth should have her blood pressure, pulse, urine output, bleeding status, and fundus checked every

BP q 2h

    a. four hours for the first 24 hours after delivery

    b. hour for the first 12 hours after delivery

    c. four hours for the first 8 hours after delivery

    d. eight hours for the first 72 hours after delivery

293   7. Occasionally, labor may bruise the urethra and bladder. The abdominal wall, weakened from pregnancy, may make urinating difficult. Catheterization may be necessary if the woman has not voided within

    a. 3 hours after delivery

    b. 6 hours after delivery

    c. 12 hours after delivery

    d. 16 hours after delivery

293   8. If a woman had a cesarean delivery, her catheter is usually removed from the bladder

    a. immediately after delivery

    b. within the first 24 hours after delivery

    c. within the first 12 hours after delivery

    d. by the third postpartum day

293   9. Early movement and ambulation after a cesarean section help with all of the following except

    a. alleviating gas pains

    b. speeding recovery

    c. decreasing venous thrombosis

    d. strengthening weakened leg muscles

293   10. The newly, cesarean-delivered mother should get out of bed briefly, assisted by the nurse,

    a. on the second postpartum day

    b. on the third postpartum day

    c. on the first postpartum day

    d. as soon as the anesthesia wears off

294   11. Colostrum provides the newborn with all of the following except

    a. immune bodies

    b. vitamin A

    c. laxity

    d. iron

294 12. Engorgement usually occurs on the second or third postpartum day and is due to all
        of the following except
        a. increased blood to the breast tissue
        b. increased lymph to the breast tissue
        c. improper latching on by the infant
        d. accumulation of milk

293 13. After a cesarean section, the incision skin sutures or clips are removed by
        a. the second postpartum day
        b. the fourth postpartum day
        c. the three-week postpartum visit
        d. dissolving on their own

294–295 14. The pain from engorgement can be relieved with all of the following measures except
        a. heat   c. a tightly fitted bra
        b. ice packs   d. manual milk expression

295 15. If a woman has sore nipples, the nurse can recommend all of the following except
        a. expressing a small amount of milk before nursing
        b. nursing more frequently for shorter periods of time
        c. offering the sore nipple first so that the baby will nurse longer on the second
            breast
        d. nursing in different positions

295 16. The let-down reflex is caused by the release of the hormone
        a. oxytocin   c. progesterone
        b. prostaglandin   d. prolactin

298 17. Postpartum depression is caused by all of the following except
        a. physiological changes that are rapidly taking place
        b. exhaustion from delivery and caring for a newborn
        c. self-doubts about abilities and the future
        d. medication given during labor

303 18. Sexual intercourse should be avoided for the first
        a. 3–4 weeks after delivery
        b. 1–2 weeks after delivery
        c. 6 weeks after delivery
        d. 8 weeks after delivery

306   19. Which of the following statements about the first few hours after delivery is true?

    a.   This is an ideal time to initiate bonding.

    b.   The baby is sleepy and not interested in his environment for the first several hours.

    c.   The mother is exhausted from labor and should be encouraged to sleep.

    d.   Baby needs immediate evaluation and mother needs to be monitored closely, so mother and baby are temporarily separated.

FILL IN THE BLANK

Complete the following statements.

289   1. The first six weeks following delivery are called the *puerperium* or the *postpartum* period.

289, 291   2. The process whereby the woman's organs return to their normal size and condition after delivery is called *involution*

290   3. During the first six weeks following delivery, the uterus changes from approximately *2* pounds to *few* ounces.

289   4. The period of the first few hours after birth is known as *4th stage*.

294   5. Milk is expected to replace colostrum in the breast tissue by the *2 or 3rd* day after delivery.

296   6. The term that refers to an infection of any part of the reproductive system after delivery is *Puerperal*.

297   7. Homan's sign is positive if there is pain behind the knee or in the calf with the leg extended and the foot flexed. A positive Homan's sign is suggestive of *Thrombophlebitis*   *puerperal thrombosis*

302   8. The average new mother will lose *18* to *20* pounds within 10 days after delivering. It is best to lose about *1/2* pound(s) per week after this until normal weight is achieved.

SHORT ANSWER

289   1. List four important principles of nursing care during the puerperium.

a. _____

_____

b. _____

_____

c. _____

_____

d. _____

_____

291–292   2. What is the purpose of afterpains?

Keeps uterus free of clots & promote involution.

299–300   3. What is the nurse evaluating when she checks the following during the postpartum period?

a. Bladder: *Urinary retention & residue urine*

b. Bowel: *Constipation*

c. Fundus: *firmness*

d. Lochia: *color, odor, amount*

e. Episiotomy: *infection – hemmorhage*

f. Breasts: *engorgement*

g. Nipples: *cracks, soreness*

293   4. List three helpful comfort measures for inflamed hemorrhoids and episiotomy pain.

a. *ice*

b. *sitz bath*

c. *oral analgesic*

cleanse area

294   5. If a woman chooses not to breast feed, what three measures can be offered to prevent or minimize milk production?

a. *Ice packs for 3 + 4 X's a day*

b. *Well-fitted bra – binder*

c. *Hormonal medication to inhibit milk & analgesic to relieve discomfort*

295   6. If a woman has a let-down sensation before she is ready to nurse, what should she be told to do to stop the flow of milk?

Press heel of hand firmly against her breasts

296   7. List three symptoms of mastitis.

a. *nausea*

b. *fatigue*

c. *Chill & fever*

296   8. Name three symptoms that suggest infection of the reproductive system after delivery.

a. *↑ T*

b. *edema*

c. *inflammation & tenderness of the part affected*

297   9. List three possible treatment measures for thrombophlebitis.

a. *↑ leg*

b. *heat cradle to protect leg*

c. *Apply dry heat*

297   10. Name three possible reasons for postpartum hemorrhage.

a. *uterine atrony*

b. *Lactation*

c. *Retainment of placenta*

298   11. List three signs or symptoms suggestive of cystitis.

a. *Painful & freq. urination*

b. *Pain over bladder*

c. *Blood purulent in urine*

Clean-catch speciment

301   12. Describe the possible menstrual cycles of a mother breast feeding her baby full time.

3 months – Nursing

7 – 9 wks – Non-nursing

Lactation influences menses & ovulation. Ovulation might be suppressed 12 - 16 months or it might begin even if there is no menses.

301–303   13. What should the nurse tell the new mother about the following at the time of discharge?

   a.   Episiotomy discomfort: _____

   _____

   b.   Elimination: _____

   _____

   c.   Flabby abdomen: _____

   _____

   d.   Diet: _____

   _____

   e.   Activity: _____

   _____

298   14. Name four signs or symptoms indicating postpartum depression.

   a. _____

   b. _____

   c. _____

   d. _____

300   15. List three things to help relieve postpartum constipation.

if ordered by Dr {
   a. *enema*

   b. *laxative*

   c. *↑ fluids & fibers*

302 16. Name six of the most common offending foods that may cause adverse reactions in the nursing infant.

  a. _____   d. _____

  b. _____   e. _____

  c. _____   f. _____

306 17. Why is the parent-infant attachment so strong during the first 30–60 minutes of life?

306 18. What are three things that can be done to help foster the parent-infant attachment?

  a. _____

  b. _____

  c. _____

MATCHING

292 Match the following terms for postpartum bleeding to the appropriate definition.

  ___3___ a. lochia alba   1. early lochia from 1st to 4th postpartum day; bright red

  ___2___ b. lochia serosa   2. lochia from the end of the first week postpartum until two weeks postpartum

  ___1___ c. lochia rubra   3. lochia from two to six weeks postpartum

Case Study

Nancy is an 18-year-old unmarried woman going home with her newborn baby. She has elected to breast feed her baby and has been successful during her hospital stay. She had no complications during her labor and delivery, and her postpartum course, so far, has been without problems. She lives with her mother and grandmother, who are both supportive and caring. Make a nursing care plan for Nancy's discharge from the hospital. Choose the most important areas to review with this 18-year-old.

CHAPTER
17
Family Planning

MULTIPLE CHOICE
Select the one best answer.

314   1. The theoretical success rate of any given contraceptive implies that the method
    a. is used correctly all the time
    b. is used correctly most of the time
    c. could be used incorrectly and accounts for errors in use
    d. is used correctly, but product defect is taken into account

314   2. When using basal body temperature (BBT) as natural family planning (NFP), instruct the woman to take her temperature
    a. as soon as she awakens after at least six hours of sleep
    b. at the end of each day
    c. anytime during the day, as long as daily recordings are at 24-hour intervals
    d. in the morning after at least eight hours of sleep

314   3. When taking the basal body temperature, which of the following indicates ovulation?
    a. temperature remains low
    b. temperature rise of $\frac{3}{10}$ to 1 degree
    c. temperature drop followed by a rise
    d. temperature rise of 1½ degrees

314   4. Natural family planning is based on the fact that
    a. ovulation occurs at midcycle
    b. ovulation occurs 14 days after the last period
    c. ovulation occurs 14 days before the next expected period
    d. the 10th to the 17th day of the month is the prime time to conceive

314, 317   5. The cervical secretions at the time of ovulation appear
   a. milky white, sticky mucus
   b. abundant, clear, slippery mucus
   c. thick, white mucus
   d. absence of mucus

314   6. Ovulation can be affected by all of the following except
   a. stress and illness   c. coitus
   b. medication   d. breast feeding

317   7. Spermicidal, to be the most effective, should be introduced into the vagina
   a. 30 minutes before intercourse
   b. 10–15 minutes before intercourse
   c. as close to intercourse onset as possible
   d. 1–2 hours before intercourse

317   8. The most common side effect(s) of spermicide is/are
   a. pregnancy   c. temporary skin irritation
   b. vaginal infections   d. pelvic cramping

318   9. All of the following about the sponge are correct except:
   a. It was approved by the FDA in 1983.
   b. It contains 1 gm of nonoxynol 9.
   c. It offers continuous protection up to 8 hours.
   d. It is disposable.

318–319   10. All of the following statements about the diaphragm are true except:
   a. It is a contraceptive barrier that creates an airtight seal against sperm.
   b. It should be inserted no more than two hours before intercourse.
   c. It has no hormonal influence on the woman's system.
   d. Some woman may experience frequent urinary tract infections.

319   11. All of the following statements about the cervical cap are true except that it
   a. was approved by the FDA in 1988
   b. grips the cervix and forms a suction
   c. may be left in place for up to five days
   d. is less messy than the diaphragm

320–321   12. All of the following statements about the IUD are correct except:
    a. It immobilizes sperm.
    b. It interferes with the endometrium.
    c. It decreases menstrual flow.
    d. It interferes with migration of sperm from vagina to fallopian tubes.

321   13. All of the following statements about oral contraceptives are true except:
    a. They are composed of estrogen and progesterone.
    b. They increase the risk of heart disease.
    c. They prevent ovulation.
    d. They offer protection against uterine and ovarian cancer.

322   14. The Norplant system consists of six silicone rods filled with
    a. estrogen   c. estrogen and progesterone
    b. progesterone   d. nonoxynol-9

322   15. The Norplant system is effective for _____ years after insertion:
    a. 3   c. 2
    b. 8   d. 5

322   16. Side effects commonly associated with the Norplant system include
    a. nausea and vomiting   c. irregular cycles and weight changes
    b. breast tenderness   d. increased cramping with menses

322   17. The Norplant system works as a contraceptive by
    a. stopping the pituitary from producing luteinizing hormone and follicle-stimulating hormone
    b. stopping the ovaries from producing estrogen and progesterone needed for ovulation
    c. changing the endometrium
    d. inhibiting sperm motility

322-323   18. The minipill differs from the combined oral contraceptive pill in all the following ways except the
    a. minipill has no pill-free days; combined oral contraceptives have seven pill-free days
    b. minipill does not consistently suppress ovulation; combined oral contraceptives suppress ovulation
    c. minipill is less effective than combined oral contraceptives
    d. absolute contraindications for combined oral contraceptives do not apply to the minipill

326   19. *Roe v. Wade* was a Supreme Court decision legalizing abortion. The ruling was made
       in

       a. 1970   c. 1975
       b. 1973   d. 1978

325   20. Depo-Provera (DMPA) 150 mg is given every_____to be an effective
       contraceptive.

       a. month   c. 3 months
       b. 2 months   d. 6 months

319   21. Women who use the diaphragm are prone to more

       a. urinary tract infections
       b. sexually transmitted diseases
       c. tissue irritation
       d. vaginal pain

FILL IN THE BLANK

Complete the following statements.

314   1. A method of natural family planning that includes checking cervical mucus and basal
           body temperature is called _____.

314–315 2. The actual success rate of natural family planning is _____ percent.

325   3. The _____ is tied in a bilateral vasectomy.

325   4. The _____ are tied in a bilateral tubal ligation.

317   5. The active ingredient in spermicides is called _____.

SHORT ANSWER

312   1. Why is it important to include the expectant father in the prenatal period?

313   2. Define the acronym BRAIDED.

    a. B: _____

    b. R: _____

    c. A:_____

    d. I:_____

    e. D:_____

    f. E: _____

    g. D:_____

314   3. Explain the difference between the actual success rate and the theoretical success rate of contraceptives.

    4. List the theoretical effectiveness rate, one advantage, and one disadvantage of each of the following contraceptives.

317   a. Spermicide: _____

            _____

            _____

318–319   b. Diaphragm: _____

            _____

            _____

319   c. Cervical cap: _____

            _____

            _____

319–320   d. Condom: _____

_____

_____

320–321   e. IUD: _____

_____

_____

320–322   f. Combined oral contraceptive: _____

_____

_____

318–319 5. Explain the major difference between the diaphragm and the cervical cap.

321 6. List four contraindications for IUD use.

a. _____

b. _____

c. _____

d. _____

320 7. Name three prerequisites for IUD insertion.

a. _____

b. _____

c. _____

321–322   8. List four possible side effects of combined oral contraceptives.

    a. _____   c. _____

    b. _____   d. _____

323   9. List nine absolute contraindications for combined oral contraceptives.

    a. _____   f. _____

    b. _____   g. _____

    c. _____   h. _____

    d. _____   i. _____

    e. _____

322   10. List four contraindications for the Norplant system.

    a. _____   c. _____

    b. _____   d. _____

325   11. What happens to the ovum after a bilateral tubal ligation?

    _____

325   12. Compare the advantages and disadvantages of a vasectomy to a bilateral tubal ligation.

    Vasectomy   Tubal Ligation

    a. _____   _____

    b. _____   _____

    c. _____   _____

    d. _____   _____

326   13. What is RU 486?

MATCHING
Match each method of contraception with the correct description of effectiveness.

314   _____   a.   natural family planning

316   _____   b.   coitus interruptus

317   _____   c.   spermicidal

318   _____   d.   sponge

318   _____   e.   diaphragm

319   _____   f.   cervical cap

319   _____   g.   condom

320   _____   h.   IUD

321   _____   i.   oral contraceptives

322   _____   j.   Norplant system

325   _____   k.   DMPA

1. lasts 24 hours and contains 1 gm nonoxynol-9

2. flexible dome-shaped device that covers the cervix and holds spermicide

3. interferes with the endometrium and the migration of sperm

4. prevents ovulation when taken daily

5. thimble-shaped device that remains in place over the cervix because of suction

6. withdrawal before ejaculation

7. nonoxynol-9 inserted intravaginally by 10–15 minutes before coitus

8. latex sheath that covers the penis

9. awareness of ovulation

10. stops pituitary gland from producing LH and FSH

11. injected every 3 months to stop ovulation

CASE STUDY

Mary is an 18-year-old, unmarried woman who has been pregnant twice. One pregnancy ended in an induced abortion. Mary's second pregnancy ended with the birth of a baby boy. Mary admits to poor compliance with barrier methods of birth control and frequently forgets to take oral contraceptives. How would you counsel Mary? What choice of birth control would you recommend for Mary? Write a brief description of BRAIDED for your recommended method of contraception so that Mary can make an informed decision.

CHAPTER
18

Characteristics and Care of the Neonate

MULTIPLE CHOICE
Select the one best answer.

331   1. Two-thirds of full term infants weigh between
   a. 2,000–2,600 gm   c. 2,500–4,000 gm
   b. 2,700–3,850 gm   d. 3,500–4,200 gm

334   2. A condition of tiny white pimples over the newborn's nose and chin is called
   a. vernix caseosa   c. infantile acne
   b. milia   d. impetigo

336   3. At birth, the eyes are blue or gray and change to their permanent color at
   a. 1 year   c. 9 months
   b. 3–6 months   d. 18 months

331   4. The average length of a newborn ranges from
   a. 18 to 22 inches   c. 19 to 21½ inches
   b. 20 to 22 inches   d. 17½ to 21 inches

333–334   5. The newborn is covered in a downy hair over the body. This is called
   a. vernix   c. lanugo
   b. milia   d. impetigo

334   6. If the baby's back is stroked on one side while the baby is lying on its stomach, the whole trunk curves to that side. This is known as the
   a. tonic neck reflex   c. placing reaction
   b. grasp reflex   d. Galant reaction

336　　7. A postural reflex in which the infant, when lying on his back, turns his head to one side and extends the arm and the leg on the side to which the head is turned at right angles from his body, is called

    a. tonic neck reflex   c. placing reaction

    b. protective reflex   d. Galant reaction

336　　8. A baby who reacts to being touched on the cheek by turning his head in the direction of the touch, is exhibiting

    a. sucking reflex   c. placing reaction

    b. rooting reflex   d. protective reflex

337　　9. All of the following procedures are performed during the first 24 hours after birth except

    a. baby's temperature is recorded

    b. baby is weighed and measured

    c. the neonatal behavioral assessment scale is given

    d. passage of urine and meconium is recorded

339　　10. The umbilical cord clamp is removed from the baby

    a. after 1 hour   c. after 24 hours

    b. after 8 hours   d. at the discharge exam

339　　11. What is needed in the baby's system before a PKU test is valid?

    a. vitamin K   c. calcium

    b. vitamin C   d. protein

340　　12. Abnormal accumulation of phenylalanine prevents

    a. normal brain development

    b. normal growth

    c. production of insulin

    d. normal respirations

341　　13. Incubators regulate all of the following except

    a. heat   c. oxygen

    b. humidity   d. light

340　　14. During the hospital stay, the nurse needs to closely supervise the baby by observing all of the following except

    a. respiration and pulse   c. Fe (iron) levels

    b. condition of cord   d. passage of urine and meconium

341   15. All of the following are used in assessing prematurity except

     a. weight

     b. gestational age

     c. behavior and appearance

     d. length

341   16. Babies who require incubators include all the following except

     a. infants weighing less than 2,500 grams

     b. infants with a positive PKU test

     c. infants who have difficulty regulating temperature

     d. infants who have respiratory difficulty

341   17. Since premature babies are susceptible to deficiency diseases, _____ may be given after the seventh day of life.

     a. antibiotics   c. extra protein

     b. vitamins and iron   d. gamma globulin

341   18. If oxygen concentrations in an incubator are over 40% for a prolonged period, it places the infant at risk for

     a. respiratory distress

     b. cyanosis

     c. blindness

     d. brain damage

344   19. The umbilical cord should be cleansed four times a day with

     a. soap and water   c. hydrogen peroxide

     b. water only   d. alcohol

341   20. The care of the premature baby includes all of the following except

     a. special feeding as needed

     b. holding and cuddling frequently

     c. weighing twice weekly

     d. wearing special gowns when handling infants

344   21. The cause of diaper rash is

     a. bacteria in urine

     b. warmth and moisture of wet diapers

     c. alkali in urine

     d. improper care of the baby

FILL IN THE BLANK
Complete the following statements.

333   1. The anterior fontanel usually closes within ____*18*____ months; the posterior
       fontanel takes ____*3*____ to ____*6*____ months to close.

334   2. The startle reflex is also known as the ____*moro*____ reflex and is a
       ____*defense*____ response of newborns.

336   3. If a reflex is absent in the newborn, it may suggest ____*CNS damage*____

341   4. The most frequent cause of death in newborn infants is ____*premature*____

SHORT ANSWER

333   1. List the normal values for the following vital signs in the full-term newborn.
       a. Temperature ____*99.5*____
       b. Pulse ____*120/150*____
       c. Respirations ____*35/50*____   *30-80*
       d. Blood pressure ____*80/46*____

333   2. Explain the law of cephalocaudal disproportion.

336   3. Name four reflexes essential to life or protection for the newborn.
       a. *Blinking*   c. *yawning*
       b *Coughing/sneezing*   d. *Swallowing/gag*

334   4. Name two purposes of the birth cry.
       a. *O2 in blood*
       b. *Expand lungs*

337   5. It is thought that the behavior of a newborn is phenotypic at birth, not genotypic.
        What does this mean?

        Both (influence) by environment & hereity

337   6. What is the major advantage of being familiar with the Brazelton neonatal behavioral
        assessment scale?

        Help in care of infants

337   7. List the four categories of behavior measured in the neonatal behavioral assessment
        scale.
        a. *social*   c. *phipical*
        b. *aclive*   d. *Stress*

339   8. Why is a vitamin K injection suggested for the newborn?

        Clotting of blood

332 9. Describe the expected appearance of a premature infant in the following categories.

   a. Weight _____

   b. Length _____

   c. Fontanel _____

   d. Features _____

   e. Skin _____

   f. Respirations _____

   g. Temperature _____

341 10. Name three areas of nursing care that need special attention when caring for the premature infant.

   a. _Airway   (O2)_

   b. _Temperature_

   c. _Adquate fluids_

342 11. List three items of information that parents should be told about circumcision of the newborn to fulfill the requirement of informed consent.

   a. _Some pain / fee_

   b. _Brief_

   c. _No legal or medical reason_

MATCHING

334, 336 Match the following reflexes with the month it is expected to disappear.

_3_ a. tonic neck reflex   1. 6th month

_2_ b. Galant reaction   2. 2nd month

_2_ c. primary standing   3. 5th month

_1_ d. Moro reflex   4. 4th month

_2_ e. automatic walking   5. as long as needed

_4_ f. grasp reflex

_5_ g. sucking reflex

_2_ h. placing reflex

EXCERCISE

Read the following procedure and be ready to demonstrate to the instructor the proper technique of bathing a new born.

Bathing the Baby:

Purpose. The infant must be given proper skin care and also should be provided comfort while being bathed. The bath experience should contribute to a loving parent-child relationship.

Precautions:

1. Always wash your hands thoroughly before starting the bath.
2. Never turn away or leave the baby alone without being sure she is secure. If it is necessary to turn away or reach for something, keep one hand on the infant to protect her from falling. If it is necessary to leave the room, pick up the infant, wrap in a blanket, and place in the crib, or carry the baby with you.
3. The room should be free from drafts. Temperature should be at least 22°–25° Celsius (72°–75° Fahrenheit).
4. Temperature of the bath water should never exceed 43° C (110° F). The general temperature range is 35°–43° C (95°–110° F).
5. Avoid chilling the infant.
6. Avoid frightening the baby. The bath should be a pleasant experience.
7. Always wash face and head first. Use clean water and washcloth.
8. Never go back to the face after changing the diaper or washing the genitals.
9. Do not oversoap the baby. A soapy baby is slippery.
10. Use long, firm, smooth strokes.
11. Pat dry to protect the tender skin; never rub dry.
12. Report any unusual changes in the skin to the doctor.

Equipment:

1. plastic tub, basin, or bathinette
2. bath mat or soft, thick towel
3. 2 towels (or 1 towel and a bath mat)
4. mild baby soap
5. cotton swabs (for cord care)
6. cotton balls
7. container for waste
8. soft washcloth
9. baby oil or cornstarch
10. diaper pail

11. baby clothes (clean shirt, diaper, gown)
12. small, cotton receiving blanket
13. crib sheets

Tub Bath:

The first six steps are the same for a sponge bath or tub bath. Usually the newborn receives a sponge bath for the first few days.

1. Wash hands and assemble equipment. Test the temperature of the bath water. It should be 35°–43° C (95°–110° F) for a tub bath.
2. Pour warm water into the plastic tub or basin. There should be no more than 3 inches of water in the tub.
3. Strip the crib to the plastic mattress covering.
4. Place the tub in a convenient location. This may be on a table or set on the crib mattress.
5. Place a towel under the infant. Have a second towel ready to cover the infant.
6. Before undressing the baby, wash the baby's face, eyes, ears, and nostrils.
   a. Using a rotary motion in the tip of the nostril, clean the nostrils with a cotton ball that has been moistened and shaped into a pledget. **Do not use cotton applicators.** Use a clean pledget for each nostril.
   b. Moisten a cotton ball. Wipe each eye away from the inner canthus (angle of eye formed by the meeting of the upper and lower eyelids closest to nose); that is, toward the outer cheek. Use a clean cotton ball for each eye.
   c. Palm the face cloth. Wash the face with clear water. Start on the forehead and make a series of Ss over and under the nose and chin. Be certain not to cover the nose and mouth at the same time, which would impair the infant's breathing.
   d. Rinse the cloth, and wash behind the ear and in the outer ear.
   e. Pat the skin dry. Rubbing irritates the skin. Be certain that the area behind each ear is clean and dry.

Sponge Bath:

The procedure for a sponge bath differs from that of a tub bath, although both start out the same way. After the face has been washed, the steps continue as follows.

1. Wash the infant's head with the specified solution and pat dry. If oil is used, be sure to remove any excess.
2. Remove the baby's shirt and diaper. If the diaper is soiled, fold the clean portion under the baby's buttocks and wash the genitals, thighs, and buttocks with cotton balls moistened with warm water. Wipe with a downward motion. Discard each cotton ball in a waste container.
3. Rinse and pat dry. Place the soiled diaper in the diaper pail. Remove the baby's shirt.
4. Cover the baby with a towel.

5. Wash neck, arms, axillae, and abdomen with solution. Give special attention to the folds of the skin. Rinse and pat dry. Cover the baby.

6. Wash the lower extremities. Pay particular attention to folds of the thighs. Rinse and pat dry.

7. Turn the infant on his abdomen and wash the back and buttocks. Rinse and pat dry.

8. Turn the baby on his back. Be sure excess oils are removed, and then dress the infant.

9. If talcum or oil is used, apply it first to your hands and then to the baby. Talcum powder tends to cake in the creases and causes irritation. Cornstarch, which is not irritating, may be used.

CHAPTER 19

Feeding the Newborn

MULTIPLE CHOICE
Select the one best answer.

350   1. The hormone responsible for milk production is
    a. oxytocin
    b. progesterone
    c. prolactin
    d. gonadotropin

350   2. Colostrum is rich in all of the following except
    a. antibiotics   c. fat
    b. salt and protein   d. iron

348   3. Emptying time of an infant's stomach varies from
    a. 1–2 hours   c. 1–4 hours
    b. 2–6 hours   d. 5 or more hours

350   4. Hormone(s) that prevent the release of milk present in the breasts during pregnancy include
    a. estrogen
    b. prolactin
    c. estrogen and progesterone
    d. progesterone and prostaglandin

351   5. Essential techniques for successful breast feeding include all of the following except
    a. proper positioning of the baby
    b. offering both breasts at each feeding
    c. proper latching on to the areola
    d. the mother's consumption of adequate milk in her diet

350   6. The success of giving an adequate supply of milk is partly dependent on

        a. the let-down reflex

        b. the size of the woman's breasts

        c. the size of the areola

        d. estrogen

351   7. The baby gets most of the milk in the first breast offered at a feeding within the first

        a. 5 minutes   c. 15 minutes

        b. 10 minutes   d. 20 minutes

354-355   8. Causes of nipple soreness include all of the following except

        a. improper latching on to the nipple

        b. restrictive feeding schedules

        c. prolonged engorgement

        d. allowing prolonged nursing time

354   9. The most critical factor in nipple soreness is

        a. the size of areola with small baby

        b. engorgement

        c. inadequate prenatal nipple preparation for nursing

        d. the latching-on technique

360   10. The breasts will continue manufacturing milk

        a. for 1 year

        b. for 18 months

        c. for 5 years

        d. indefinitely with stimulation and correct hormone balance

348   11. The method that works best for successful breast feeding is

        a. scheduled feeding times

        b. demand feeding

        c. supplementing with water

        d. supplementing with formula

354   12. Smoking can cause all of the following effects to a mother's milk supply except

        a. reduction of milk production

        b. reduction of vitamin C concentration

        c. respiratory problems for the infant

        d. diarrhea and colic in the infant

353   13. When breast feeding a baby, a woman's diet must be monitored in all of the
        following ways except

    a. quality of food   c. increased fluid intake

    b. quantity of food   d. increased milk intake

354   14. A woman requires _____ milligrams of calcium above her maintenance needs
        to breast feed while she is pregnant.

    a. 800 mg   c. 600 mg

    b. 1,200 mg   d. 400 mg

359   15. If the infant fails to gain weight, and seems fussy, frustrated, and hungry after an
        adequate period of time at the breast, the most likely cause is

    a. allergy to the milk

    b. inadequate milk supply

    c. breast infection

    d. reaction to a food the mother may have eaten

360   16. All of the following situations are reasons why a woman should not breast feed
        except

    a. breast reduction

    b. the mother has hepatitis

    c. the mother has HIV

    d. breast augmentation

360–361 17. The best way to wean a baby is to

    a. stop offering the breast when weaning is desired

    b. stop nighttime breast feeding first

    c. gradually eliminate one feeding at a time and substitute with formula

    d. bottle feed the baby when he is hungry, and breast feed only for comfort so the
        supply and demand production of milk decreases naturally

FILL IN THE BLANK

Complete the following statements.

351   1. Both breasts should be offered at each feeding as emptying the breasts stimulates

    _____ and prevents _____ .

352   2. Milk stored in the alveoli and milk-producing cells of the breast is called

    _____Hinde_____ ; milk stored under the nipple that is not as rich in fats
        and calories is called _____Fore_____ .

358   3. The most prominent symptom of a clogged duct is

_____ .

358   4. A generalized soft tissue infection in the breast is called _____ .

362   5. When a tube is placed into the baby's stomach via his nose or mouth for the purpose

of feeding, it is called _____ feeding.

SHORT ANSWER

350   1. List four reasons, other than hunger, that cause a baby to cry.

a. _____   c. _____

b. _____   d. _____

348   2. Briefly define feeding on demand.

_____

351   3. Explain how fear, pain, or other stresses physiologically affect breast feeding.

351–352   4. Name three indications that confirm the baby is getting enough milk.

a. _____

b. _____

c. _____

351–352   5. Briefly describe proper positioning and breast feeding techniques as you would if teaching a new mother.

354   6. List three reasons why breast feeding is recommended.

    a. _____

    b. _____

    c. _____

354–355   7. Name five possible causes for some nipple soreness.

    a. _____

    b. _____

    c. _____

    d. _____

    e. _____

355–356   8. List five interventions to decrease sore nipples in the breast feeding woman.

    a. _____

    b. _____

    c. _____

    d. _____

    e. _____

357–358   9. List five interventions to help alleviate engorgement pain.

a. _____

b. _____

c. _____

d. _____

e. _____

356   10. Name three ways to stimulate flat nipples to a more erect state to facilitate latching on by the infant.

a. _____

b. _____

c. _____

358   11. List three interventions to alleviate a plugged duct.

a. _____

b. _____

c. _____

359   12. List four interventions to help correct an inadequate milk supply in the breast feeding mother.

a. _____

b. _____

c. _____

d. _____

359–360   13. Name five nursing interventions that will soothe a fussy baby.

a. _____

b. _____

c. _____

d. _____

e. _____

360   14. What can a mother do to make breast feeding more comfortable for herself after a cesarean birth?

a. _____

b. _____

360   15. Define weaning.

360–361 16. Explain how you would instruct a new mother to wean her baby.

361–362 17. Name three principles that are important to teach a new mother about bottle feeding her infant.

    a. _____

    b. _____

    c. _____

363–364 18. Describe the use of a Lact-Aid.

Disorders of the Neonate

Multiple Choice

Select the one best answer.

368 1. All of the following characteristics of the newborn's respiratory system are accurate except:

    a. It normally has a slightly irregular pattern.

    b. Respirations vary from 40–60 per minute.

    c. It normally is regular in pattern.

    d. Spontaneous breathing occurs within 30 seconds after birth.

369 2. All of the following symptoms are common to respiratory distress syndrome except

    a. cyanosis

    b. a loud cry in attempts to get air

    c. dyspnea

    d. nasal flaring

369–370 3. The criteria evaluated in the Silverman-Anderson Index include all of the following except

    a. chest lag and intercostal retraction

    b. xiphoid retraction and nasal dilatation

    c. expiratory grunt

    d. respirations per minute

370 4. Jaundice can be caused by all of the following except

    a. breast milk

    b. failure of liver to breakdown red blood cells

    c. hemolytic disease

    d. anoxia

371   5. The most common treatment for jaundice is
- a. phototherapy
- b. none needed
- c. medication
- d. transfusion

373   6. The major problem with a cleft palate and cleft lip is
- a. appearance
- b. breathing difficulty
- c. feeding difficulty
- d. risk of infection

374   7. The signs of pyloric stenosis include all of the following except
- a. dehydration
- b. a mass felt in the right upper quadrant of the abdomen
- c. a protrusion in the abdominal wall
- d. poor skin turgor

374   8. Colic is most likely to occur during the
- a. first year of life
- b. first 6 months of life
- c. first 3–4 months of life
- d. first 6 weeks of life

374   9. To treat diarrhea in the newborn, the mother should be instructed to do all of the following except
- a. limit formula feedings
- b. give 5% glucose in saline solution every 3–4 hours until the diarrhea subsides
- c. contact the baby's physician
- d. stop breast feeding completely

374   10. Symptoms suggesting pyloric stenosis first appear
- a. within a few hours after birth
- b. 2 to 4 weeks after birth
- c. when the baby is weaned
- d. when the baby starts solid foods

374   11. The treatment for pyloric stenosis is
- a. to restrict solid foods
- b. no treatment is necessary
- c. surgical
- d. medication

381   12. Phenylketonuria is a metabolic disorder caused by failure of the body to oxidize
       phenylalanine causing problems to the
       a. digestive system
       b. circulatory system
       c. brain
       d. lymphatic system

378   13. The risk for the development of a Down syndrome infant at age 40 is
       a. 1:885   c. 1:109
       b. 1:12   d. 1:85

379   14. Abnormal turning of an infant's foot or feet is termed
       a. torticollis   c. talipes
       b. Erb's palsy   d. congenital dislocation

379   15. The shortening of the sternocleidomastoid muscle is called
       a. torticollis   c. talipes
       b. Erb's palsy   d. congenital dislocation

379   16. A damaged brachial plexus is called
       a. torticollis   c. talipes
       b. Erb's palsy   d. congenital dislocation

380   17. Neonatal hypothermia is more commonly seen in
       a. infants who are small for their gestational age
       b. infants with respiratory distress syndrome
       c. infants who are large and born to diabetic mothers
       d. Down syndrome infants

381   18. In the infant, glycogen is stored at higher-than-adult concentrations in all of the
       following organs except the
       a. liver   c. heart
       b. skeleton   d. pancreas

382   19. When the urethra terminates on the underside of the penis, it is called
       a. hermaphroditism
       b. hypospadias
       c. epispadias
       d. exstrophy

382   20. The integumentary system of the newborn includes all of the following except
       a. epidermis   c. hair and nails
       b. teeth buds   d. corium layer

FILL IN THE BLANK
Complete the following statements.

368 1. Deprivation of oxygen in the newborn is called *anoxia* .

370 2. In the Silverman-Anderson Index, a score of *0* indicates no respiratory distress; a score of *10* indicates severe respiratory distress.

371 3. When a baby's red blood cells are destroyed by Rh antibodies, it results in a condition called *erythroblastosis fetalis* . This condition is uncommon today because of the gamma globulin medication called *RhoGAM*

373 4. A fissure in the roof of the mouth and nasal cavities is called a *cleft plate* .

373 5. Thrush is an infection caused by a *Candida (fungus)*

384 6. Another name for miliaria rubra is *prickly heat.*

385 7. Impetigo is a serious skin infection and is caused by *Staphylococcal*

384 8. Cellular or vascular local anatomic alterations of the skin are called *nevi* .

371 9. RhoGAM is administered *3* days after delivery.

SHORT ANSWER

368 1. Name three ways a nurse can offer support to parents who have delivered an infant with a physical or mental disease.

a. _____
b. _____
c. _____

368 2. Name three conditions that can produce anoxia in the fetus.

a. _____
b. _____
c. _____

369 3. Describe the cause of respiratory distress syndrome.

368   4. Define congenital disorder.

_____

369   5. Name two symptoms of respiratory distress syndrome.

    a. _____

    b. _____

369   6. What is the Silverman-Anderson Index?

_____

369   7. List five principles of care to follow when treating a baby who does not breathe
      spontaneously at birth.

    a. _____   d. _____

    b. _____   e. _____

    c. _____

370   8. What causes physiological jaundice in the newborn?

381   9. List six signs or symptoms associated with low blood sugar levels in the newborn.

    a. _____   d. _____

    b. _____   e. _____

    c. _____   f. _____

371   10. When an infant's red blood cells are being destroyed by Rh antibodies, what
       symptoms are carefully monitored by the health team?

    a. _____   c. _____

    b _____   d. _____

374–375 11. Name three symptoms of imperforate anus.

    a. _____

    b. _____

    c. _____

378   12. Define hydrocephalus.

380
382   13. Define pseudohermaphroditism.

*Newborn has external sex organs
of 1 sex & gonads of other sex*

385   14. Describe the difference between cephalhematoma and caput succedaneum.

MATCHING

Match the following neural tube defects with the correct definitions.

376   __2__   a. spina bifida occulta   1. spinal cord and meninges protrude through defect in the spinal canal

376   __3__   b. meningocele   2. defect only in the vertebrae

376   __1__   c. meningomyelocele   3. meninges protrude through the opening in the spinal cavity

EXERCISE

Explain how to resuscitate a newborn, who has no heart beat and is not breathing, without the use of hospital equipment.

CASE STUDIES

1. Sarah and Joe delivered their first son, and he was diagnosed with imperforate anus. What symptoms would lead health providers to suspect imperforate anus? What is necessary to correct this anomaly? What should the nurse tell Sarah and Joe about their son's prognosis?

2. Jan delivered her fourth daughter, who was immediately diagnosed with cleft lip and cleft palate. At what point during pregnancy did this defect occur? What are the health implications for this baby? What can be done to correct the anomaly? What special care will the parents need from the health care team?

CHAPTER 21

Principles of Growth and Development

MULTIPLE CHOICE
Select the one best answer.

391   1. The continuous and complex process in which the body and its parts increase in size is known as
    a. development
    b. growth
    c. differentiation
    d. integration

391   2. The qualitative and continuous process by which the child's level of functioning and progression of skills become more complex is known as
    a. development
    b. growth
    c. differentiation
    d. integration

392   3. The process by which maturation begins at the head and moves downward to the toes is known as
    a. cephalocaudal
    b. integration
    c. proximodistal
    d. sequential

393   4. The pace of growth and development is
    a. standardized
    b. varied
    c. nonsequential
    d. uncertain

393   5. The progression from general responses to more skilled responses is known as
    a. growth
    b. development
    c. differentiation
    d. integration

393 6. A 4-year-old throws a ball using no footwork, and a 12-year-old throws a ball with precise footwork. This is an example of
   a. growth
   b. development
   c. differentiation
   d. integration

393 7. A 2-year-old uses one or two words for a sentence, and a 10-year-old uses many words for a sentence. This is an example of
   a. integration
   b. development
   c. differentiation
   d. hierarchy

394 8. Bone structure and adult height are affected most by
   a. environment
   b. learning
   c. heredity
   d. integration

394 9. To foster growth and development parents should begin to provide stimulation during the
   a. toddler stage
   b. neonatal stage
   c. infant stage
   d. school stage

394 10. One of the primary reasons for the nurse to know principles of growth and development is to provide
   a. a schedule for visiting hours
   b. a care plan adapted to the needs of the child
   c. a list of favorite toys of the child
   d. the ability to work with the health care team

FILL IN THE BLANK

Complete the following statements.

392 1. Infants control the movements of their ___hands___ before they control their ___feet___ movements.

392 2. Before an infant can touch an item, he first can ___gaze___ at it only.

393 3. The rate of growth for the fetus and infant is ___rapid___. After the age of 12 months growth ___slows___ and then progresses at a ___steady___ rate.

393 4. Infants have *large* heads compared to the rest of the body.

394 5. In children who are malnourished, growth may be *retarded*.

393 6. A 20-month-old child can jump in *place*, and a 7-year-old can jump *rope*.

393 7. *Integration* is the ability to develop simple skills and functions into higher order skills and functions.

394 8. To foster growth and development, *A stimulating environment* is an important part of the process and must be provided by parents and caretakers.

SHORT ANSWER

394 1. List three factors that influence growth and development.
   a. *Social*
   b. *economic*
   c. *educational*

391 2. Define five principles of growth and development.
   a. _____
   b. _____
   c. _____
   d. _____
   e. _____

394 3. List three reasons why it is important for nurses to know principles of growth and development.
   a. _____
   b. _____
   c. _____

MATCHING

Match the term in the left column with their definitions in the right column.

391	_9_ a. growth	1. simple skills and function to higher order skills and functions
393	_1_ b. integration	2. level of functioning more complex
391	_2_ c. development	3. begins at center of body outward toward the extremities
393	_10_ d. sequential	4. from general responses to more skilled responses
392	_8_ e. cephalocaudal	5. genetic factors
393	_4_ f. differentiation	6. from simple to complex tasks
393	_6_ g. hierarchal integration	7. socioeconomic
384	_5_ h. heredity	8. begins at head and proceeds downward
291–292	_3_ i. proximodistal	9. body and parts increase in size
394	_7_ j. cultural environment	10. events occur in a patterned and predictable manner.

CASE STUDIES

1. A mother asks you in the well baby clinic why her 11-month-old child is not walking yet. His brother walked at 10 months.
   a. Explain how growth and development vary with each child
   b. Explain to the mother the developmental sequence that occurs before the child can walk.

2. You are assigned to a day care center. You will be working in the infant unit. In the area, you have four children between 11 and 14 months. Observe the behavior and report on the following: eye-hand coordination, motor development, and speech. Describe similarities and differences.

CHAPTER

22

Physical Growth

MULTIPLE CHOICE
Select the one best answer.

398   1. The most rapid period of growth occurs during
    a. adolescence   c. toddler age
    b. preschool   d. infancy

399   2. The average infant's birth weight will be tripled by
    a. 3 months   c. 9 months
    b. 12 months   d. 6 months

399–400   3. At birth, baby Ann was 20 inches long. On her third birthday, she will be
    a. 43–45 inches long
    b. 32–34 inches long
    c. 37–39 inches long
    d. 47–49 inches long

400   4. The fastest-growing part of a child during childhood is the
    a. arms   c. trunk
    b. legs   d. head

399   5. The period between infancy and adolescence in which physical growth slows and stabilizes is
    a. toddler age   c. preschool
    b. school age   d. adolescence

400   6. The familiar awkwardness of childhood is most pronounced during
    a. toddler age   c. school age
    b. puberty   d. adolescence

400   7. During the period of adolescence, the teenager gains what percentage of final adult weight?
    a. 30%   c. 50%
    b. 25%   d. 75%

400   8. During adolescence, the reproductive organs double in size under the hormonal influence of the

     a. thyroid gland   c. parathyroid gland

     b. pituitary gland   d. pancreas gland

402–403   9. The number of deciduous teeth a 1-year-old will have is approximately

     a. 12   c. 6

     b. 9   d. 3

402–403   10. The permanent teeth emerge at about 6 years. The number will be

     a. 24   c. 28

     b. 20   d. 32

FILL IN THE BLANK

Complete the following statements.

398   1. In infancy, very rapid growth occurs between __birth__ and __1__ year(s) of age.

399   2. The period between infancy and preschool is called __toddler__.

399   3. The trunk of a toddler has a characteristic __potbelly__ appearance.

400   4. Fat tissue increases slowly until approximately the age of __7__.

400   5. The average age of puberty is between 9½ and 14½ in __girls__.

400   6. The principal sign of sexual maturity in boys is the presence of __sperm__ in the urine.

400   7. __Menstruation__ signals the onset of sexual maturity in girls.

402   8. Skeletal growth is complete when the __growth__ plate of the __long__ bones of the arms and legs have completely __fused__.

402   9. Skeletal growth is complete in girls at age __15½__ and boys at age __17½__.

403   10. The name given to the first teeth is __deciduous__ __primary__.

SHORT ANSWER

Describe the changes in physical growth during

398-399 infancy   Height: _____

Weight: _____

399–400 preschool   Height: _____

Weight: _____

399-400 school age   Height: _____

Weight: _____

400 adolescence   Height: _____

_____

Weight: _____

_____

MATCHING

Match the terms in the left column with their definition ins the right column.

398–399	__4__ a. infancy	1. teeth begin to erupt
399	__5__ b. toddlerhood	2. slow, steady growth during this period
403	__1__ c. deciduous teeth	3. characterized by development of sex characteristics
399–400	__7__ d. preschool	4. very rapid growth and development
399–400	__2__ e. school	5. slower growth during this period
401	__3__ f. adolescence	6. onset of sexual maturity in girls
403	__8__ g. permanent teeth	7. physical growth slows and stabilizes
400	__6__ h. menstruation	8. teeth erupt at age 6

ACTIVITIES

400 1. You are assigned to prepare a class for adolescent boys and girls.

Have the students describe how they feel about their bodies. This should be a written exercise first, and then students can discuss it openly if they want. Explain to the students how their bodies are being affected by hormones and what physical and emotional changes are occurring.

398 2. You are assigned to give a prenatal class to mothers on the first year of an infant's life. Describe normal growth during the first year.

CASE STUDIES

1. Mrs. Smith has three children ages 2, 5, and 10. She comes to the doctor's office with the children's height and weight charts and records. She wants you to explain why there is a difference in each child's results. Compare the charts with Mrs. Smith, and explain that there is a normal range of height and weight.

2. You are working in a dental office, and a mother brings in her 4-year-old child. The child fell off her bike and broke her front tooth. The mother says, "Well, it really won't matter—these were only her baby teeth." Explain to the mother the importance of good dental care and how it affects the permanent teeth.

Developmental Stages

MULTIPLE CHOICE
Select the one best answer.

407 1. Which phrase best defines personality?
   a. unique individual with different growth patterns
   b. a person's style of approaching others
   c. pattern of characteristic thoughts that distinguishes one person from another
   d. pattern of growth that demonstrates a different developmental pattern

407–408 2. The way in which a person approaches people and life situations is called
   a. differentiation
   b. temperament
   c. personality
   d. integration

408–409 3 Freud's theory of personality development is also known as
   a. conflict resolution
   b. psychosocial
   c. intellectual development
   d. psychosexual

408 4. According to Freud, the ego part of the personality represents
   a. conscience
   b. reason or common sense
   c. shoulds and should nots
   d. the pleasure principle

408, 410   5. The theory of psychosocial development has been developed by
- a. Freud
- b. Piaget
- c. Kohlberg
- d. Erikson

410   6. A key phrase associated with Erikson's theory of psychosocial development is
- a. pleasure principle
- b. learning trust
- c. nurturing experience
- d. moral reasoning

408   7. That particular challenge must be resolved at each stage of development in order for healthy personality to develop is a theory of
- a. Freud
- b. Kohlberg
- c. Erikson
- d. Piaget

410   8. A child saying "no" demonstrates a sense of autonomy that usually occurs at the age of
- a. birth to 1 year
- b. 1 to 3 years
- c. 4 to 6 years
- d. 6 to 12 years

408   9. The theory of intellectual or cognitive development was developed by
- a. Kohlberg
- b. Piaget
- c. Erikson
- d. Freud

411   10. According to Piaget, a child can reason well if concrete objects are used. This reasoning usually occurs at the age of
- a. 2 to 7
- b. 4 to 7
- c. 7 to 11
- d. 11 to adult

408   11. Kohlberg's theory of development is called
- a. psychosexual development
- b. moral development
- c. psychosocial development
- d. cognitive development

408–409   12. The stage at which there is an internalized standard of behavior on which to base decisions is known as the
- a. trust vs. mistrust stage
- b. preconventional stage
- c. conventional stage
- d. postconventional stage

409   13. Examples of gross motor skills would include all except
- a. throwing a ball
- b. crawling
- c. holding a crayon
- d. standing alone

412   14. At the age of 3 years, according to the Denver Developmental Screening Test in language development, the child should be able to do all but
- a. name one picture
- b. speak understandably at least 50% of the time
- c. name four colors
- d. combine words

426   15. The literal meaning of words is most significant to the
- a. infant
- b. preschooler
- c. school-age child
- d. teenager

FILL IN THE BLANK
Complete the following statements.

407–408   1. Differences in temperament remain _consistent_ as the child grows older.

408   2. Freud's theory of _____ development focuses on the shift of gratification from ____/____ body _zone_ to the next.

408   3. Erikson's theory of personality development is divided into _____ stages of _____ span.

410   4. According to Erikson, the final stage of development that occurs between 12 and 18 years is known as _____ vs. _____ .

411   5. Symbols are used to represent objects, according to Piaget, during the _____ stage, which occurs between ____2____ and ____4____ years.

TRUE OR FALSE

426   _T___ 1. As a person goes through adolescence, he will experience an increase in dexterity as well as increased awkwardness.

426   _T___ 2. The adolescent relates to peers rather than parents.

426   _F___ 3. The adolescent unconditionally accepts traditional values of the parents.

425   _F___ 4. The adolescent experiences a growth spurt and a decrease in strength.

426   _F___ 5. The adolescent develops emotional maturity during the teen years.

THE STORY OF HOPE

Write the missing words to complete the story.

Hope was born on October 3, 1980.

She was 9 lb., a little bit over weight.

415   At the age of _____ month(s), she could hold her hand in a _____

She was able to smile, and when prone turn her _____ a little _____ .

416   Hope at four months rolled from _____ to _____ ,

Played with her fingers and followed you with her eyes.

416   She put objects in her mouth at _____ months of age.

416   With her arms for support, she _____ on the floor as if it was her stage

417   Now, at the age of _____ months, she can _____ without support.

417   Her first words were _____ and _____ , we must report.

418   The world now becomes bigger as Hope begins to _____ about the floor.

418–419   And _____ to Mommy as she says "Stay away from the door."

Hope has now reached the age of one

And her age of independence has just begun.

ACTIVITIES

420   1.   For a 15-month-old child describe:

       a.   two gross motor skills

Walk

Crawl

       b.   two fine motor skills

feed self

Hold a cup

422   2. For a 2-year-old child describe:

       a.   two fine motor skills

Draw a picture

Use crayons

       b.   four language skills

300 words - talks a lot

Knows name

411   3.   You are addressing the parents of toddlers. Describe how you would use anticipatory guidance to assist in preparing a child for pre-K.

424   4.   You will be speaking to a group of 8-year-old boys and girls about a physical education program. Name the age-appropriate activities you would have them do.

CHAPTER

24

𝒩utrition

MULTIPLE CHOICE
Select the one best answer.

433   1. The major nutrients necessary for body functions are
    a. fats, lipids, protein, minerals, and vitamins
    b. carbohydrates, starches, fats, minerals, and vitamins
    c. carbohydrates, protein, fats, minerals, and vitamins
    d. carbohydrates, protein, vegetables, fats, and minerals

433   2. The major source(s) of ready energy is/are
    a. carbohydrates   c. fats
    b. protein   d. minerals

436   3. A major food group necessary to build and repair tissue is
    a. carbohydrates   c. fats
    b. proteins   d. minerals

436   4. Symptoms of lack of protein would include all but
    a. skin patches and scales
    b. shiny, colorful hair
    c. edema
    d. muscle wasting

437   5. The essential minerals for normal bone and tooth development are
    a. calcium and sodium
    b. calcium and phosphorous
    c. calcium and potassium
    d. calcium and magnesium

439   6. Solid foods are added at about 4–6 months; new foods should be introduced one at a time at intervals of

      a. 3–5 days   c. 1 week

      b. 2 weeks   d. 3 weeks

441   7. Toddlers, because of their rapid growth, are at a risk of

      a. rickets

      b. dental caries

      c. bruising

      d. iron-deficiency anemia

443   8. A lunch that would be appealing and nutritious for an 8-year-old could be

      a. slice of pizza and milkshake

      b. peanut butter sandwich, potato chips, and milk

      c. hamburger, french fries, and milkshake

      d. tacos, french fries, and milkshake

443   9. The caloric intake for an adolescent should be

      a. less than an 8–12-year-old

      b. more than an 8–12-year-old

      c. less than a 4–8-year-old

      d. more than a 4–8-year-old

438   10. The food pyramid recommends the following servings

      a. bread and cereal 6–11; meat 2–3; fruit 2-4

      b. bread and cereal 2–3; meat 2–3; fruit 2-4

      c. bread and cereal 2–4; meat 2–3; fruit 6-11

      d. bread and cereal 6–11; meat 2–3; fruit 3-5

FILL IN THE BLANK
Complete the following statements.

433   1. Two important factors that influence the selection of food are _____ and

      _____.

433   2. An inadequate intake of essential nutrients results in _____ .

433   3. Prolonged carbohydrate deficiency can lead to _____ damage.

436   4.   Fats are made up of _____ , which consist of three fatty acids and

_____.

439   5.   Breast milk is recommended for infants because it is less likely to cause food

_____ and contains maternal _____ .

442   6.   Toddlers like to use the same spoon and fork. This is known as

_____ .

SHORT ANSWER

439   1.   List five points to teach parents regarding infant's diet and nutritional needs.

     a. _____
     b. _____
     c. _____
     d. _____
     e. _____

442   2.   List three points to teach parents about a preschooler's diet.

     a. _____
     b. _____
     c. _____

443   3.   List three points to teach parents about a school-age child's diet.

     a. _____
     b. _____
     c. _____

MATCHING

Match the terms in the left column with their definitions in the right column.

437   _____a. vitamin A   1.   found in plant sources

436   _____b. complete protein   2.   aid in energy metabolism

437   _____c. fluoride   3.   helps eyes to adjust to dim light

436   _____d. incomplete protein   4.   prevents dental caries

437   _____e. B complex   5.   found in animal sources

ACTIVITIES

435 1. Plan a breakfast for a family of Chinese national origin.

436 2. You are assigned to a Head Start day care center. Decribe what you would expect to look for as signs of malnutrition in a 4-year-old.

CHAPTER

25

$\mathscr{I}$mmunizations

MULTIPLE CHOICE
Select the one best answer.

448   1. The single most important event that prevents communicable disease in children is
    a. the discovery of antibiotics
    b. genetic screening
    c. immunization programs for children
    d. prenatal classes for pregnant women

448   2. An immune response occurs when white blood cells are stimulated to produce antibodies. These are called
    a. monocytes   c. neutrophils
    b. lymphocytes   d. eosinophils

448   3. Active immunity occurs when individuals form antibodies against specific diseases by
    a. transferring of antibodies from mother to child
    b. getting the infectious disease
    c. receiving antibodies from someone who has had the disease
    d. receiving gamma globulin

449   4. The American Academy of Pediatrics' Committee on Infectious Disease recommends that immunizations begin at
    a. 2 months   c. 3 months
    b. 2 years   d. 6 years

449   5. The recommended immunization schedule for children at 6 months include
    a. MMR, DTP, HB   c. DTP, HiB, HB
    b. MMR, DTP, HB   d. MMR, DTP, OPV

451   6. Children over the age of 7 years may experience adverse reactions if they receive the

        a. HB vaccine   c. DTP vaccine

        b. MMR vaccine   d. DT vaccine

450   7. An allergy to eggs would prevent vaccination for

        a. hemophilus influenza

        b. diphtheria,tetanus, pertussis

        c. measles, mumps, rubella

        d. polio

451–452   8. Recently in the U.S. there has been as increase in rubeola cases; therefore, the following immunization schedule is recommended

        a. 15 months, 6 years

        b. 12 months, 3 year

        c. 5 months, 10 years

        d. 2 months, 2 years

452   9. Babies may be born blind, deaf, or develop heart disease if the mother during her pregnancy contracts

        a. rubeola   c. hepatitis B

        b. rubella   d. mumps

452   10. A swelling of the parotid glands may be the result of vaccination with

        a. OPV   c. MMR

        b. HB   d. DTP

FILL IN THE BLANK
Complete the following statements.

448   1. As of 1977, the U.S. Department of Health and Human Services began a childhood *immunization* program.

448   2. An individual becomes resistant to a disease through a process called *immunity*

448   3. A child may receive ready-made antibodies from someone else. This type of immunity is called *passive*   .

STUDENT'S NAME: _____

448   4. A _*toxoid*_ is an active immunizing agent that is made up of an infectious antigen.

449   5. A vaccination may not provide lifelong immunity; therefore, vaccines need to be given periodically. This is known as a _____ shot.

450   6. A DTP vaccine means the child will have immunity to _____ , _____ and _____ .

450, 451   7. If someone in the household is immunosuppressed because of AIDS or cancer therapy, the child should not receive _OPV_ _____ vaccine.

451   8. A major cause of meningitis and bacteremia in children under the age of five is _*Hib*_ .

452   9. Before a vaccination is given to a child, the parent must sign an _*consent*_ .

454   10. Vaccination should be postponed if a child has a _*fever*_ .

SHORT ANSWER

448   1. List and describe three forms of vaccines.
   a. _____
   b. _____
   c. _____

449   2. Name the nine infectious disease for which a vaccine is available.
   a. _____   f. _____
   b. _____   g. _____
   c. _____   h. _____
   d. _____   i. _____
   e. _____

453–454   3. Prepare a sample of a child's health record. Include the following information.
   Date of immunization: _____
   Vaccine: _____
   Manufacturer and batch number: _____
   Site and route of administration: _____
   Name and title of person giving vaccine: _____

MATCHING

Match the terms in the left column with their definitions in the right column.

451   _3_ a. DTP

451   _5_ b. polio *ATDS*

451   _1_ c. HiB

452   _2_ d. HB

451   _4_ e. MMR

1. redness and swelling at injection site

2. few reactions

3. fever of 104°F, persistent cry

4. rash and fever

5. contraindicated with immunosuppressed children

CASE STUDIES

1. As many as 50% of children under the age of two are not immunized. You are assigned to a well-baby clinic. A mother comes in with her 15-month-old son. You ask her about the baby's immunizations. She states that she does not believe in vaccinations. Discuss how to educate her on the benefits of this program.

2. As part of your maternity clinical rotation, you must give a class to new mothers on the importance of immunizations for their infants. Prepare a chart on the immunization for the first year of life and the diseases they prevent.

Explain why it is important to keep all records regarding immunization schedules.

Child Safety

MULTIPLE CHOICE
Select the one best answer.

458   1. Knowledge of child development is critical to prevent
    a. birth defects
    b. vitamin deficiency
    c. communicable disease
    d. accidents

460   2. Federal regulations cover all of the following except
    a. proper restraints for children in automobiles
    b. use of flame-retardant fabric for children's sleepwear
    c. safety caps on children's prescriptions
    d. storage of household cleaners in the house

460   3. The most common pediatric emergency is
    a. falls   c. car crashes
    b. poisoning   d. burns

464   4. After sudden infant death syndrome, the second leading cause of death in infants under 6 months of age is
    a. drowning   c. suffocation
    b. child abuse   d. accidents

464   5. A child who would be at a risk for child abuse may have any of the following characteristics except
    a. middle child   c. slow learner
    b. chronic illness   d. physical disability

465   6. The correct way to assist breathing in an infant is to
    a. form a mouth seal with no pinching of the victim's nose
    b. place your mouth over the infant's mouth and nose, creating a seal
    c. place your mouth over the infant's nose, pinching the lips
    d. form a mouth seal pinching the victim's nose

467   7. To check for circulation in children, palpation of the _____ is recommended.

      a.   radial artery

      b.   brachial artery

      c.   temporary artery

      d.   carotid artery

infants brachial artery

467   8. Rescue breathing in an infant should be done at the rate of _____ breaths per minute.

      a.   10

      b.   20

      c.   30

      d.   40

467   9. The compression for children in CPR is

      a.   ½–1 inch at the rate of 80 breaths per minute

      b.   ½–1 inch at the rate of 100 breaths per minute

      c.   1–1½ inches at the rate of 80 breaths per minute

      d.   1–1½ inches at the rate of 100 breaths per minute

468   10. In children under one year of age, the Heimlich maneuver is a combination of

      a.   five back blows and five chest thrusts

      b.   five back blows and four chest thrusts

      c.   four back blows and five chest thrusts

      d.   six back blows and six chest thrusts

FILL IN THE BLANK

Complete the following statements.

459   1. The number one cause of death in children is the result of *accident*

460   2. In cases of poisoning, further absorption may be prevented by syrup of ipecac, gastric lavage, or *activated charcoal*

460   3. Syrup of ipecac is used to induce *vomiting* .

460   4. Parents should be instructed that syrup of ipecac should take effect within *15* to *20* minutes.

460   5. Child abuse includes physical abuse, emotional abuse, verbal assault, and

464

Sexual assault.

465 6. The three basic skill groups of cardiopulmonary resuscitation are known as the ABCs of CPR. These include _Air_ , _Breathing_ and _circulation_

468 7. The most common cause of respiratory distress in children is _air obstruction_

468 8. The size, shape, and _consistency_ of an object swallowed by a child, determine the degree of danger to the child.

468 9. When using the Heimlich maneuver with children, use _sub diaphrag_-abdominal thrusts. _make_

MATCHING
Match the term in the left column with the definition in the right column.

462 __5__ a. gastric lavage

464 _____ b. child abuse

464 __1__ c. physical abuse

__8__ d. neglect

465 _____ e. resuscitation

464 __4__ f. emotional abuse

467 __3__ g. brachial artery

465 __9__ h. CPR

468 __7__ i. Heimlich maneuver

464 _____ j. sexual abuse

1. deliberate injury to the body

2. child's participation was obtained by force or gifts

3. checkpoint of pulse for CPR

4. interaction that causes psychological pain

5. instilling large amounts of water in the stomach

6. restoring to life

7. abdominal thrusts used to open blocked airways

8. deliberate lack of care for child's basic needs

9. cardiopulmonary resuscitation

10. an intentional physical or emotional mistreatment

SHORT ANSWER

461   1. List the six steps for a safety checkup on a car seat.

a. _____

b. _____

c. _____

d. _____

e. _____

f. _____

462   2. Name three developmental factors that place toddlers at risk for poisoning.

a. _____

b. _____

c. _____

EXERCISES

1. Demonstrate CPR for an infant and a child on an anatomical model.
2. Demonstrate the Heimlich maneuver for an infant and child on an anatomical model.

CASE STUDIES

1. Juan, who is 18 months old, is brought to the emergency room by his mother. He has fallen down the front steps. Juan's mother states she "doesn't know what to do—he is always having accidents." Explain to the mother how to prevent falls, burns, poisoning, and other possible accidents in a toddler.

2. A father calls the emergency room and states he is not able to rouse his 12-year-old son. There is a bottle of pills nearby. What information must you obtain from the father?

3. Jimmy, age 3, is a patient in the pediatric unit. He was admitted with suspicious bruises and burn marks on his buttocks. Johnny's father is suspected of child abuse. His mother comes to visit Johnny. How would you initiate a therapeutic conversation with this parent?

CHAPTER

27

Preparing for Hospitalization

MULTIPLE CHOICE
Select the one best answer.

473   1. Hospitalization of a child creates stress for all family members. To reduce stress, the nurse can plan all the following except
   a. preadmission activities
   b. a family visit to the lab
   c. discharge planning
   d. day-of-admission activities

473   2. To further reduce stress, the nurse may
   a. have the family select the type of diet for the child
   b. allow family members to tour the hospital
   c. give an orientation to the family about the daily routine at the hospital
   d. give the sick child permission to watch television all day

474   3. To reduce anxiety and build trust, the best response to family's questions regarding the illness could be:
   a. "Since children are young and healthy in general, they recover quickly."
   b. "Dr. Smith has been taking care of this type of illness for a long time."
   c. "Tell me what you know about the illness, and I will try to explain it."
   d. "Look around here. The children don't really seem that sick, do they?"

474   4. The mother comes to you and says, "I don't understand. Samantha stopped sucking her thumb two years ago and has started again." Your best response would be
   a. "Tell Samantha she's a big girl now, and thumb-sucking is for babies."
   b. "It's a normal reaction when children are frightened. Children sometimes resort to thumb-sucking when they are frightened of something."
   c. "Would you like me to put a bandage on that finger?"
   d. "We'll just ignore it. I'm sure it won't happen again."

474   5. Preadmission preparation should include all but
   a. honest and accurate information
   b. enough time between sessions for parents to formulate questions
   c. assessment of parents' resources to pay for services
   d. consideration of language or cultural barriers

476   6. An appropriate toy for a preschool child would be
   a. stuffed animals
   b. coloring books and writing material
   c. a telephone
   d. doctor and nurse puppets

476   7. Adolescents should be told about their hospitalization about
   a. 1–3 days prior to admission
   b. as soon as the need is determined
   c. 4–6 days prior to admission
   d. 1 week prior to admission

477   8. An activity to help reduce trauma of hospitalization for a school-age child would be to
   a. explain in simple terms how they will feel better
   b. introduce the child to the unit and the room
   c. allow the child to handle the equipment
   d. involve the child in planning care

477   9. The biggest fear of preschool children regarding hospitalization is
   a. having needles stuck in them   c. separation from parents
   b. loss of identity   d. the inability to visit with peers

473   10. A critical element to assess how a family will react to the child's illness is to
   a. know the cultural background of the family
   b. understand growth and development
   c. determine the economic status of the family
   d. observe the interaction between family members

FILL IN THE BLANK
Complete the following statements.

473   1.   The recent trend in hospital care of children includes _____.

473   2.   It is important for the nurse to stress to parents the idea that they are an
             _____ part of the recovery process.

473   3.   One of the most frequent coping mechanisms parents use is _____.

477   4.   Separation anxiety is greatest for the _____.

475   5.   One area of teaching that is often neglected is the impact of hospitalization on the
             _____ of the hospitalized child.

SHORT ANSWER
477   Name six stressors that affect a child's hospitalization.

             a. _____

             b. _____

             c. _____

             d. _____

             e. _____

             f. _____

Assessment

MULTIPLE CHOICE
Select the one best answer.

757   1. When Margaret, age 6 months, came to the pediatric clinic, she was weighed. Her birth weight was 9 lb. Her current weight should be
- a. 12 pounds
- b. 15 pounds
- c. 18 pounds
- d. 21 pounds

482   2. Indicators of physical growth in a child include all but
- a. height
- b. chest circumference
- c. temperature
- d. weight

484   3. When using an oral thermometer, you must leave it in place for _____ minutes.
- a. 2
- b. 1
- c. 4
- d. 3

484   4. Before taking an oral temperature, the nurse must assess if the child has a history of
- a. impetigo
- b. cystic fibrosis
- c. PKU
- d. convulsions

484   5. Which is the least stressful way to take the temperature of a 3-year-old?
- a. oral
- b. tympanic
- c. rectal
- d. axillary

486 6. The normal heart rate range for a 7-year-old is _____ beats per minute.
   a. 80–130
   b. 70–120
   c. 70–110
   d. 60–100

486 7. An important consideration when taking a child's blood pressure is the
   a. size of the cuff
   b. size of the child
   c. use of a mercury or electronic device
   d. weight of the child

485 8. Children may have a normal cycle of irregular rhythm associated with respirations. This is called
   a. sinus bradycardia
   b. sinus arrhythmia
   c. sinus rhythm
   d. sinus tachycardia

FILL IN THE BLANK
Complete the following statements.

486 1. A vital-sign assessment of a child includes temperature, pulse, respirations, and

_____.

482 2. When placing an infant on a scale, it is important to remember to place a

_____ on the scale to prevent _____ from touching the baby's skin.

484 3. A child's temperature can be measured through an oral, axillary, rectal, or

_____ route.

484 4. The length of time a rectal thermometer is kept in place is _____ to

_____ minutes.

484–485 5. The _____ pulse is preferred on children under the age of 5.

ACTIVITIES

1. You were requested to prepare a class for preschool parents on normal growth and development. Complete the following chart to show normal findings for 3 to 5-year-olds.

482   Height:_____   Weight:_____

484   Temperature: _____   Pulse: _____

486   Respirations:_____   Blood pressure:_____

484 2. List the devices used to measure temperature in children, and state how long they must be kept in place for an accurate reading.

a._____

b._____

c._____

CHAPTER

29 | *The Hospitalized Child*

MULTIPLE CHOICE
Select the one best answer.

490   1. Separation anxiety begins when children are about the age of
    a. 4 months   c. 6 years
    b. 8 months   d. 8 years

491   2. Jane, age 2, has been admitted to the pediatric unit with pneumonia. Her mother leaves for the admission office, and Jane crawls into a corner of the youth bed. Jane is demonstrating
    a. protest
    b. separation anxiety
    c. despair
    d. detachment

491   3. A toddler may exhibit protest by
    a. thumb-sucking
    b. withdrawal
    c. attacking strangers by hitting them
    d. being less demanding

492   4. Kenneth is 2½ years old. He is able to drink water from a cup. When he is admitted to the hospital, he wants a bottle. This is an example of
    a. denial   c. regression
    b. repression   d. suppression

494   5. Margaret is 12 years old and must be admitted to the hospital. The best way to help Margaret adjust would be to provide a

     a. telephone   c. VCR

     b. television   d. compact disc player

494   6. Allowing the young patient to sleep late and not be awakened for early morning routines would be most beneficial to which age group?

     a. toddler   c. school-age child

     b. teenager   d. infant

496   7. Fear of not getting well is most prevalent with

     a. infants   c. school-age child

     b. toddler   d. adolescent

496–497   8. Doing a procedure in the treatment room rather than the child's room is most helpful to decrease anxiety for

     a. the adolescent   c. the infant

     b. the toddler   d. all of the above

497   9. Danny is 7. He has to have his broken arm set and casted. The best way to explain the procedure is by

     a. having him read a story

     b. using diagrams, models, and equipment

     c. allowing him to participate in the decision making

     d. allowing him to visit the operating room

   10. Nurses can help parents cope with a child's hospitalization by

     a. supporting family members

     b. providing information

     c. preparing for discharge and home care

     d. all of the above

FILL IN THE BLANK

Complete the following statements.

490   1. Stressors of hospitalization for children of all ages include _____ ,
loss of _____ , fear of _____ , and _____ .

490   2. Parents are encouraged to stay with children and _____ in their care.

492   3.   School-age children may benefit most from _____ activity during hospitalization to reduce stress.

495   4.   Appropriate pharmacologic pain-control measures should be used for children of _____ age groups.

496   5.   The fear of losing all their blood after an injection is most common in the _____ age group.

ACTIVITIES

492–493   1.   Vincent, age 3, has to go to the hospital. Explain to the parents what type of behavior to expect. Name the toys appropriate for this age group. Describe three ways you can assist Vincent in maintaining control.

495–496   2.   Describe how the following age groups would react to pain.

Infant: _____

_____

Preschooler: _____

_____

School-age child: _____

_____

Adolescent: _____

_____

CHAPTER
30

Routine Pediatric Procedures

MULTIPLE CHOICE
Select the one best answer.

502 1. Factors the nurse must consider to prepare a child for procedures include all except
- a. economic status
- b. age
- c. developmental stage
- d. ability to reason

502 2. While under the care of the baby sitter, Jamie, age 6, falls and breaks her arm. Jamie is taken to the emergency room. To obtain an informed consent, the doctors should
- a. have Jamie's brother, age 20, sign the consent
- b. not worry about consent; it is an emergency
- c. call the parents and obtain a verbal consent; two people must document the verbal consent
- d. have the baby sitter sign the consent since she was left in charge

503 3. The best restraint for 18-month-old Michael, who is having a repair of a harelip deformity, is
- a. elbow restraint
- b. papooose board
- c. mummy restraint
- d. wrist restraints

505   4. While holding and transporting an infant, the nurse must rest the baby's head and neck in the palm of the hand. This is known as the
    a. upright hold   c. football hold
    b. transport hold   d. cradle hold

506   5. In administering liquid medication to an infant, you may use all the following except a
    a. calibrated dropper
    b. medicine cup
    c. bottle with formula
    d. plastic syringe

507   6. Tommy is 5 months old. To give him an intramuscular injection, the recommended site is the
    a. deltoid muscle
    b. vastus lateralis muscle
    c. dorsogluteal muscle
    d. gluteus maximus muscle

507   7. Jo-Ann, age 6, has otitis media. You must place ear drops into her ear by pulling the pinna
    a. down and back   c. up and back
    b. down and front   d. up and front

511   8. When a tracheostomy must be suctioned, the nurse must proceed with the catheter by going in suction port
    a. closed, coming out suction port open
    b. open, coming out suction port closed
    c. closed, coming out suction port closed
    d. open, coming out suction port open.

510   9. Nasogastric tubes are used for all the following reasons except to
    a. provide liquid feedings for a child who refuses to eat
    b. provide liquid feedings for a child who cannot swallow
    c. decompress the stomach
    d. lavage the stomach

513   10. When giving a gavage feeding, the nurse should have the child's bed in the following position
    a. semi-Fowler's   c. Fowler's
    b. supine   d. Trendelenberg

FILL IN THE BLANK
Complete the following statements.

503   1.   Infants are usually placed in a _____ crib to protect them from injury.

503   2.   When applying elbow restraints to a child, the nurse must place the armboard on the _____ side of the arm.

505   3.   To position a child for a lumbar puncture, the nurse must be certain that when holding the child in the correct position, the _____ is not interfered with.

507   4.   One of the dangers in giving medication to a crying child is _____.

507   5.   Instilling eye medication, the nurse should pull the lower lid, and place the eye ointment into the _____ conjunctival sac starting from the _____ canthus.

510   6.   A _____ tube is surgically placed in the stomach for long-term feedings.

MATCHING
Match the terms in the left column with their definitions in the right column.

502   _____   a.   Infant   1.   may fear bodily harm; use the language of the child

502   _____   b.   Toddler   2.   acts stoic while maitaining self control

503   _____   c.   Preschooler   3.   give pacifier or bottle

503   _____   d.   School-age child   4.   provide distraction

503   _____   e.   Adolescent   5. procedure may be feared as punishment

ACTIVITIES

503   1.   Outline the procedure for the use of a papoose board.

506   2.   List the five rights of giving medications.

a. _____

b. _____

c. _____

d. _____

e. _____

507   3.   In assessing an IV infusion, you must check for

a. _____

b. _____

c. _____

d. _____

CHAPTER 30

4. Select the correct word from the word list to fill in the blanks.

nasal cannula	stay	diagram	saliva
face mask	doll	forearm	burette
medicine cup	gloves	femoral vein	infusion pump
urine	oxygen	orally	intramuscular

Mary Jane is admitted to the hospital with pneumonia. She is 4 years old. The nurse requests that the parents _____ . On admission, the laboratory technician must draw blood. To help relieve anxiety, the technician gives Mary Jane a _____ to explain the procedure. Mary Jane watches while the technician washes his hands, puts on _____ , and then draws the blood from her _____ .

The nurse comes into the room to start an IV with antibiotics. To ensure the proper rate of flow, the medication is administered through a(n) _____ . To help Mary Jane breathe, the nurse helps her put on a funny _____ through which _____ will flow.

After three days, Mary Jane's temperature is down, and the doctor says she is ready to go home. You should instruct the parent to give medication _____ by a _____. The nurse gives Mary Jane a hug for being a good patient and tells her parents to be sure to call the doctor if Mary Jane has a temperature again.

CHAPTER

31

The Pediatric Surgical Patient

MULTIPLE CHOICE
Select the one best answer.

517 1. One of the reasons for the change from inpatient to outpatient surgical settings is
   a. hospitalization causes lasting psychological stress
   b. reduced risk of infection
   c. the recovery time is shorter
   d. it reduces health care costs

519 2. To relax the child before going to the operating room, the nurse may do all of the following except
   a. orient the child to unfamiliar surroundings
   b. place the child in a quiet room with the parents
   c. include family members in preop teaching
   d. allow the child to keep all his clothes on

521 3. The purpose of preparing the operative site is to
   a. remove all pathogenic organisms
   b. keep tape from sticking to the skin
   c. decrease the chance of infection
   d. make the area more visible to the surgeon

520 4. Preparing a child for a surgical procedure by allowing her to view a film in which peers model behavior is best suited for
   a. a toddler   c. a preschooler
   b. an adolescent   d. a school-age child

524   5. The nurse must check the preop checklist for all of the following except
        a. allergies noted on the chart
        b. vital signs obtained and recorded
        c. an electrocardiogram
        d. mouth checked for loose teeth

525   6. A change in a child's behavior postoperatively is most indicative of
        a. fear and anxiety
        b. postoperative pain
        c. the need for fluids
        d. discomfort from the intravenous

525   7. To relieve pain without medication, the nurse might say all of the following except:
        a. "I'll rub your back."
        b. "Go to sleep, and the pain will disappear."
        c. "Take a deep breath, and slowly let it out."
        d. "I'll get Mommy and Daddy to stay with you for a little while."

527   8. Careful disposal of diapers helps
        a. to make the child more comfortable
        b. to prevent diaper rash
        c. to reduce the risk of infection
        d. in measuring urinary output

529   9. To be certain the child is in fluid balance postoperatively, the nurse should do all except
        a. measure food and fluid intake
        b. record intake and output record
        c. weigh the diapers
        d. weigh the child daily

FILL IN THE BLANK
Complete the following statements.

524   1. The nurse must be sure to check the chart for a _____ informed consent before the operation.

527 2. The child should be kept NPO according to the doctor's order preoperatively because of the fear of _____.

524 3. Before the nurse gives any preop medication, she must identify the patient by checking the _____.

524 4. When a child is transferred from the postanesthesia room to her room, the report must include the patient's status, what occurred during surgery, and if any _____ was given postoperatively.

525 5. To help assess the quality of the child's postoperative pain, the nurse might use the _____ rating scale.

527 6. To decrease the chance of aspiration, the child should be kept _____ until _____ sound returns.

529 7. To promote healing, the nurse must be certain that a _____ appropriate diet is given.

SHORT ANSWER

517 1. List the six stressors that produce anxiety for the child and parents during surgery.

a. _____   d. _____

b. _____   e. _____

c. _____   f. _____

525 2. List at least six nonpharmacological methods to assist with pain control in the care of the pediatric patient.

a. _____   d. _____

b. _____   e. _____

c. _____   f. _____

518–521;
526–529
Susan is 5 years old and is admitted with chronic otitis media. She is scheduled for a myringotomy. Prepare a nursing care plan for Susan's preoperative and postoperative care. For each problem, establish a goal and four nursing interventions that are specific for Susan.

Problem	Goal	Nursing Interventions
Anxiety related to surgery		
Potential injury resulting from surgery		
Potential for inadequate hydration		
Parents are not knowledgeable regarding illness		

CHAPTER

32

Caring for the Dying Child

MULTIPLE CHOICE
Select the one best answer.

535   1. One of the greatest challenges facing nurses is helping a family care for
    a. a chronically ill child
    b. a child who becomes paralyzed
    c. a child with muscular dystrophy
    d. a dying child

535   2. The concept of death, or non-life, begins at the age of
    a. 12 months   c. 3 years
    b. 2 years   d. 6 years

536   3. The statement least likely to be made by school-age children who are seriously ill is:
    a. I know I will be better in heaven.
    b. Leave me alone. I don't want to play.
    c. I'm not going to take the medicine. I hate it.
    d. I hate all the doctors and nurses.

537   4. Which of the following statements demonstrate the dying child is in a state of bargaining?
    a. I will be going home tomorrow to play with my friends.
    b. I hate my sister and her friends.
    c. If I eat all my vegetables and take my medicine, I will grow up to be big and strong.
    d. Where I am going, I won't be in pain.

193

5. Johnny is terminally ill. The reaction least likely to come from his parents is:

   a. Johnny will get his treatment and be better.

   b. If I took Johnny to the doctor sooner, this wouldn't have happened.

   c. This is the way life is, and we must accept it.

   d. I don't care what you say—you don't know how to take care of my son.

6. Nursing information for the care plan of a dying child includes all but

   a. the current health status of the child

   b. the stage of grieving of the family

   c. plans for the integration of school work

   d. how siblings are reacting to the child's impending death

7. Susan, age 10, may feel better about her brother's critical illness if she is permitted to

   a. talk to her friends about her brother

   b. continue with her own activities

   c. visit the hospital and play with her brother

   d. clean the house for her parents

8. Which of the following could be the most supportive for the entire family unit of a terminally ill child?

   a. Ronald McDonald house

   b. pediatric unit of the hospital

   c. hospice care

   d. participating in a Make-a-Wish activity

9. Hospice care includes which of the following?

   a. diagnostic testing

   b. pain control measures

   c. radiation therapy

   d. surgical intervention

10. When caring for a dying child, the nurse may experience

    a. isolation from the family unit

    b. ambivalence

    c. extreme protectiveness toward the child

    d. guilt over own feelings

FILL IN THE BLANK
Complete the following statements.

535   1. One of the most common events in which a child may see death occur is when a
_____ dies.

535   2. A 5-year-old might believe she can make anything happen. This process is
called _____ .

536   3. The school-age child tends to think that death is caused by their
_____ or _____ .

537   4. The _____ becomes emotionally attached to doctors or nurses
during a life-threatening illness.

538   5. The process whereby parents begin to work through accepting the loss of their child
is known as _____ .

539   6. Nurses who care for a child who is dying must first examine their own
_____ .

540   7. Allowing parents and siblings to express feelings is a plan of action that addresses
the problem of _____ .

541   8. To allow a dying child to express his feelings reduces his _____ and
_____ .

540   9. To help a family cope with the child's illness, the nurse may ask the parent to
_____ the child's care.

539 , 540   10. Another measure of comfort for family members is _____ support.
Nurses should be certain to allow patients and their families _____ .

MATCHING
Match the terms in the left column with their definitions in the right column.

535   _____ a. 6 months   1. expresses some appropriate grief
535   _____ b. 2 years   2. loss of control
535   _____ c. 3 years   3. unaware of death
536   _____ d. 6 years   4. magical thinking
536   _____ e. 9 years   5. speak to person who died
536   _____ f. 15 years   6. death is seen as a ghost

ACTIVITY

536-537;
540-542 You have been asked to admit Gerard, who is 14 years old. Gerard is diagnosed with cystic fibrosis and is extremely ill. Write a nursing care plan to reduce anxiety for patient and family. Be aware of Gerard's stage of development and how to meet his psychosocial needs.

Problem	Goal	Nursing Intervention
Anticipatory grieving		
Fear and anxiety		
Loss of peer status		
Loss of control		

CHAPTER

33

Sudden Infant Death Syndrome

MULTIPLE CHOICE
Select the one best answer.

546 1. The other name for sudden infant death syndrome is
   a. crib death
   b. prenatal death
   c. neonatal death
   d. infant death

546 2. The cause of SIDS is
   a. bacterial pneumonia
   b. viral pneumonia
   c. unknown
   d. hyaline membrane disease

546 3. SIDS occurs more frequently in
   a. spring between midnight and 9 A.M.
   b. winter between midnight and 9 A.M.
   c. spring between 9 A.M. and midnight
   d. winter between 9 A.M. and midnight

546 4. The recommended position for healthy infants to sleep is
   a. prone position
   b. semi-Fowler's position
   c. supine position
   d. Fowler's position

547 5. A family has just had an infant die from SIDS. The nurse can help the family by doing all except
   a. suggest the family have another baby
   b. give the parents the baby's footprints
   c. allow the parents to hold the infant
   d. provide privacy for all members of the family

FILL IN THE BLANK
Complete the following statements.

546   1.   The leading cause of death in children between 1 and 12 months is

_____.

546   2.   The most common racial group in which SIDS occurs is

_____.

546   3.   The color of mucus usually found with infants with SIDS is

_____ , frothy fluid from the nose and mouth.

547   4.   In the case of an unexplained death, most states require an _____

to determine the cause of death.

547   5.   The name of the support group for SIDS parents is

_____.

ACTIVITIES

546   1.   Describe the pattern of risk factors for SIDS.

547   2.   The parents found their baby dead and have brought the child to the emergency room.
Explain how you will approach the parents. Describe what their feelings might be.
How can you relieve their anxiety?

CHAPTER 34

Communicable and Infectious Diseases

MULTIPLE CHOICE

Select the one best answer.

553   1. The best definition of communicable disease is

    a. disease that is caused by an antigen-antibody reaction

    b. disease that is spread from one person to another either directly or indirectly

    c. disease that is caused by pathogenic viruses that invade the body, reproduce, and multiply

    d. disease that is caused by microorganisms that invade the body, reproduce and multiply

553   2. In the chain of infection, the way in which the organism leaves the reservoir is known as the

    a. portal of entry

    b. portal of exit

    c. susceptible host

    d. transmission

554   3. Disease can be spread in all of the following ways, except by

    a. the air   c. heredity

    b. an indirect host   d. direct contact

554   4. The incubation period is best described as the period

    a. that begins when a pathogen invades the body and ends when the disease process begins

    b. that begins when the body is infected by a pathogen and ends when the person starts to shed the pathogen

    c. that follows the incubation period

    d. that begins when the latent period ends and continues as long as the pathogen is present

5. To minimize the risk of exposure to the blood and body fluids of all patients, the best method of infection control is

   a. handwashing; use of mask and gloves

   b. use of gown and gloves; handwashing

   c. isolation of all contaminated linen

   d. universal precautions

6. One cause of AIDS in children may be

   a. siblings with AIDS

   b. a pediatrician who treats AIDS patients

   c. amniotic fluid or mother's milk

   d. commercial milk products

7. Oatmeal baths are a treatment for

   a. rubella   c. herpes

   b. chicken pox   d. rubeola

8. The initial signs of Lyme disease in children is

   a. a red rash called erythema migrans

   b. a macular, papular rash

   c. a three-stage rash

   d. Koplik spots on the buccal mucosa

9. The incubation period for rubeola is

   a. 10–21 days   c. 5–7 days

   b. 10–12 days   d. 5–21 days

10. The Epstein-Barr virus is the causative agent in

   a. rubella

   b. Lyme disease

   c. Fifth disease

   d. mononucleosis

FILL IN THE BLANK

Complete the following statements.

1. Communicable diseases must be reported to the ___local health Dept.___ .

553   2. The process of the development of infectious disease is called the

Chain of infection

554   3. A critical element to prevent disease is _Infection control_.

555   4. The purpose of isolation is to prevent the _transmission_ of the disease.

557   5. The time from exposure to the AIDS virus and illness in children may be up to _10_ years. The tragedy of AIDS is there is no _cure_.

SHORT ANSWER

553   1. Name the three major causes of disease.
    a. _bacteria_
    b. _viruses_
    c. _parasites_

553–554   2. List the links in the chain of infection.
    a. _Agent_   _transmission_
    b. _reservoir_   _Port of entry_
    c. _portal of exit_   _host_

554   3. Name the four identifiable stages of infection.
    a. _latent_
    b. _incub_
    c. _Comm._
    d. _disease_

555–556   4. List the most important techniques used in isolation. _Private room_
    a. _Wash hands_
    b. _gloves_
    c. _gown_
    d. _mask_
    e. _equipment_
    f. _needle safety_
    g. _Containment articles Double bag_

Integumentary Conditions

MULTIPLE CHOICE
Select the one best answer

572　1. The skin performs all the following functions except
    a. protects against the sun
    b. acts as a waterproof covering
    c. is an organ of sensation
    d. is an organ of circulation

572　2. Another name for the hypodermis layer is:
    a. epidermal layer
    b. subcutaneous layer
    c. cutaneous layer
    d. dermal layer

575　3. This condition of infants is seen more in warm weather than in cool weather.
    a. eczema
    b. diaper dermatitis
    c. miliaria rubra
    d. atopic dermatitis

575　4. An inflammation of the skin caused by a primary irritant or allergen contact is called
    a. seborrheic dermatitis
    b. diaper dermatitis
    c. atopic dermatitis
    d. contact dermatitis

576   5. In this inflammation of the skin, which occurs in childhood, the lesion is typically scaly, dry, thickened, and pruritic. This condition is known as

      a. contact dermatitis   c. impetigo

      (b.) eczema   d. miliaria rubra

577   6. A highly contagious bacterial infection of the skin is

      a. eczema   (c.) impetigo

      b. ringworm   d. tinea pedis

582   7. Direct contact with flame or hot liquids causes a/an

      (a.) thermal burn

      b. chemical burn

      c. electrical burn

      d. radiation burn

583–584   8. A partial thickness burn is also known as

      a. superficial   c. first degree

      (b.) second degree   d. third degree

586   9. The most common fear of children and parents with burns is

      a. infection   c. disfigurement

      b. treatment   (d.) pain — *drsg chang*

583–585   10. Burn wound care includes all the following except

      a. hydrotherapy

      (b.) skin traction

      c. surgical excision of eschar

      d. application of burn dressing

FILL IN THE BLANK

Complete the following statements.

572   1. Effective treatment of skin conditions often requires the child to receive treatment over a ___*long*___ period of time.

573   2. Miliaria rubra also is called ___*prickly heat*___ because the rash creates a ___*prickling*___ or ___*stinging*___ sensation.

575   3. If a diaper rash lasts more than 4 days, the causative organism is
       Candida albicans (monilia

576   4. Another name for seborrheic dermatitis is *Dandruff - Cradle ca*

577   5. Characteristic round lesions with central clearing and a scaly border is known as
       Ringworm .

578   6. Mothers fear their children will come home from school with the condition known as
       Pediculosis Capitis   . The most common symptom is itching.
       lice

581   7. The lesion found in type 1 herpes, which occurs on the upper or lower lip, is called a
       Cold sore   .

586   8. A split thickness graft that is removed from an unburned portion of the child's body
       and placed on the open wound is called a(an) *autograft* .

SHORT ANSWER

575–577   1. Name five skin conditions that affect infants and toddlers. Describe their causes and
       treatment.

Disease	Cause	Treatment
a. *Miliaria Rubra*		
b. *Contact Dermatitis*		
c. *Diaper Dermatitis*		
d. *Eczema*	*allergy hereditary*	
e. *Dandruff*		

577–578 2. Name four classifications of ringworm. — *fungal*

puselofel VIN (left margin)

   a. *Tinea capites - scalp (Kerion)*
   b. *Tinea corporis - ringworm*
   c. *" " cruris - jock itch*
   d. *" " pedis - foot*

583 3. List the factors involved in evaluating the classification and severity of burns.
   a. *Type of burn*
   b. *depth*
   c. *duration of contact*   *Lund Browder*

586 4. List four common topical burn medications.
   a. *Silvadeen*   c. *Aqueous silver nitrate*
   b. *Sulfamylon*   d. *Povidone-iodine*

586 5. Name and describe the three types of skin grafts.
   a. *Allograft - cadaver*
   b. *Xenograft - pigskin*
   c. *Autograft - own from epidermis + dermis.*

MATCHING
Match the terms in the left column with their definitions in the right column.

	Lesions			Definitions
574	*5*	a.	plaque	1. raised red spot on surface of the skin
574	*6*	b.	wheal	2. pus-filled, raised area
574	*9*	c.	macule	3. collection of dead serum
574	*10*	d.	patch	4. fluid-filled, raised area
574	*1*	e.	papule	5. raised, thickened portion of the skin
574	*2*	f.	pustule	6. elevated area, irregular shape
574	*4*	g.	vesicle	7. excess dead epidermal cells
574	*8*	h.	bulla	8. fluid-filled, raised area larger than 1 cm
574	*7*	i.	scale	9. a flat spot, flush with skin surface, different in color
574	*3*	j.	crust	10. flat surface tissue, differs from surrounding skin in color and texture

CASE STUDIES

1. A mother brings her 3-year-old child to the doctor and states, "I think my daughter is allergic to cotton. There is a rash around her ankles." Name the condition and describe the treatment to the mother.

   The mother is worried her daughter's friends won't play with her. What important role does the nurse play in discussing skin conditions with the mother?

2. Describe the psychosocial impact of acne on the adolescent. How would you counsel a teenager with this condition?

3. Tommy, age 7, was helping his Dad light the barbecue. There was an explosion, and Tommy received severe burns to 30% of his lower body. You must develop a nursing care plan that includes the physical, emotional, and social impacts of this accident.

Problem	Nursing Intervention
Potential for shock	
Hypovolemic shock	
Potential for infection	
Pain	
Fear and anxiety	

Conditions of the Eyes and Ears

MULTIPLE CHOICE
Select the one best answer.

591　1. Symptoms of strabismus or misalignment of the eyes may include
   a. myopia
   b. presbyopia
   c. diplopia
   d. amblyopia

591　2. If Carolyn, age 2, has trouble picking up blocks from the floor, you may suspect she has
   a. conjunctivitis
   b. strabismus
   c. cataract
   d. glaucoma

592　3. A clouding of the lens that prevents light from reaching the retina is called
   a. glaucoma   c. amblyopia
   b. strabismus   d. cataracts

592　4. Children who exhibit symptoms of this communicable condition are generally sent home from school. This condition is known as
   a. cross-eyes   c. cataracts
   b. pinkeye   d. tearing of the eyes

594   5.   Color vision testing should be performed between the ages of
        a.   2 months and 2 years
        b.   2 years and 4 years
        c.   4 years and 8 years
        d.   8 years and 12 years

596   6.   Infants and children are more prone to otitis media than adults because the eustachian tube is angled
        a.   more horizontally
        b.   less horizontally
        c.   more vertically
        d.   less vertically

596   7.   Objective signs of otitis media will include all except
        a.   crying
        b.   pulling at the ear
        c.   pain in the ear
        d.   drainage from the ear

597   8.   To prevent future occurrences of otitis media, the nurse should instruct the parents to
        a.   prop the infant for feeding
        b.   place infants in upright position for feeding
        c.   allow infant to take bottle to bed
        d.   restrict visitors from seeing infant

FILL IN THE BLANK
Complete the following statements.

591   1.   In strabismus, the eyes may turn inward (_____), outward (_____), upward (_____), or downward (_____).

592   2.   Children usually are tested before preschool for this condition known as _____, or lazy eye.

593   3.   An injury to the eye that may occur on the ski slope could be an ultraviolet _____ of the _____ .

596   4.   Inflammation of the middle ear is known as _____ .

597   5.   Hearing is assessed by _watching_ children's reaction to

_____ stimuli.

MATCHING
Match the terms in the left column with their definitions in the right column.

591	_3_	a. photophobia	1. eyes turning inward	
591	_6_	b. strabismus	2. refractive ability	
597	_10_	c. myringotomy	3. sensitivity to light	
591	_9_	d. diplopia	4. wearing a patch over eye	
591	_8_	e. visual acuity	5. pink eye	
596	_7_	f. tympanometry	6. misalignment of the eye	
597	_5_	g. conjunctivitis	7. measurement of the internal ear pressure	
592	_4_	h. occlusion therapy	8. area of vision	
591	_1_	i. esotropia	9. double vision	
594	_8_	j. visual field	10. surgical incision of ear drum	

CHAPTER 37

Cardiovascular Conditions

MULTIPLE CHOICE
Select the one best answer.

601
1. Heart disease that occurs during fetal development is known as
   a. cyanotic heart disease
   b. congenital heart disease
   c. acquired heart disease
   d. acyanotic heart disease

602
2. The structures that enable the blood of the prenatal infant to bypass the liver and lungs include all but
   a. foramen ovale
   b. ductus venosus
   c. pulmonary artery
   d. ductus arteriosus

603
3. The majority of congenital heart disease develops during the
   a. first 4 weeks of fetal life
   b. 4th through 12th weeks of fetal life
   c. 7th through 12th weeks of fetal life
   d. 4th through 7th weeks of fetal life

603–604
4. Some of the most common heart diseases caused by congenital defects are all but
   a. transposition of the great vessels
   b. patent ductus arteriosus
   c. rheumatic heart
   d. tetralogy of Fallot

605   5. A continual flow of blood from the aorta to the pulmonary artery occurs in the congenital condition known as

      a. patent ductus arteriosus
      b. transposition of the great vessels
      c. atrial septal defect
      d. patent foramen ovale

607   6. The symptoms of a full, bounding pulse in the upper extremities with a weak pulse in the lower extremities occurs in the condition known as

      a. patent ductus arteriosus
      b. pulmonary stenosis
      c. coarctation of the aorta
      d. ventricular septal defects

610–611   7. The initial goal of therapy in the treatment of congestive heart failure is to

      a. maintain the heart rate at 80
      b. decrease the need for oxygen
      c. increase urinary output
      d. correct the congenital defect that caused CHF

611   8. Hypertension in children is diagnosed when the

      a. systolic or diastolic pressure is above the 95th percentile for the age and sex on more than three visits
      b. systolic or diastolic pressure is above the 85th percentile for the age and sex on more than three visits
      c. systolic or diastolic pressure is above the 95th percentile on more than one visit
      d. systolic or diastolic pressure is above the 95th percentile on more than five visits

616   9. The Jones criteria used to diagnose rheumatic fever includes

      a. carditis, polyarthritis, chorea
      b. carditis, polyarthritis, clubbing
      c. carditis, hypertension, chorea
      d. carditis, polyarthritis, cardiomegaly

614   10. The most common acquired heart disease in children is

      a. hypertension
      b. congestive heart disease
      c. rheumatic heart disease
      d. pulmonic stenosis

FILL IN THE BLANK
Complete the following statements.

603   1. The foramen ovale closes within a _Several wks_ after birth.

603   2. The ductus arteriosus can _reopen_ under stressful conditions such as _hypoxemia_.

603   3. No change in skin color is noted in _Acyanotic_ heart disease.

610   4. In the aftercare of a patient with a cardiac catherization, it is most important for the nurse to check the extremities for capillary filling time, _Color_, _temperature_ and _sensation_.

608   5. Clubbing of the fingers and toes may be a symptom of the congenital heart defect known as _Complete t of Great Vessels_

611   6. The drug of choice to treat congestive heart failure is _Digoxin_. Be certain to check the _Pulse_ before administering the drug.

611   7. The room of the child with CHF should be _neutral thermic_, and the bed should be in _Semi - Fowler_ position.

614   8. The most common site in the heart affected by rheumatic heart disease is the _mitral_ valve. The disease frequently occurs 2–3 weeks after a _A beta strep_ infection.

615   9. Chorea is characterized by _involuntary_, rapid movements of the _face_ and _limbs_.

616   10. The treatment for rheumatic disease is to give the child _antibiotic_ for a period of _10_ days.

MATCHING

Match the terms in the left column with their definitions in the right column.

615   __10__   a.   chorea   1. ventricular septal defect

603   __4__   b.   cyanotic heart disease   2. cardiac catheterization

611   __8__   c.   tachycardia   3. echocardiogram

603   __1__   d.   acyanotic heart disease   4. tetralogy of Fallot

603   __2__   e.   invasive procedure   5. pulmonic stenosis

610   __7__   f.   left ventricle unable to pump   6. enlarged liver

609   __9__   g.   hypoxemia   7. congestive heart failure

603   __3__   h.   noninvasive procedure   8. rapid heart rate

607   __5__   i.   valvotomy   9. diminished oxygen

       __6__   j.   hepatomegaly   10. St. Vitus dance

ACTIVITY

609–612   Victoria is 9 months old. Her parents bring her to the pediatric clinic. They state that Victoria turns blue when she starts to crawl, she isn't gaining weight, and she is very sleepy. After an initial examination, the doctor schedules a cardiac catheterization. He tells the parents that Victoria has a heart condition known as tetralogy of Fallot, and her condition can be improved by a surgical procedure.

As the primary nurse assigned to Victoria, do the following:

a.   Describe a cardiac catheterization.

b. To relieve anxiety, describe to the parents how the normal heart functions and what occurs in the tetralogy of Fallot. Use diagrams to describe both conditions.

c. Describe the surgical procedures that will correct the condition.

d. List at least four nursing interventions to assist both patient and family to relieve stress.

CHAPTER 38

Respiratory Conditions

MULTIPLE CHOICE
Select the one best answer.

621   1. The exchange of oxygen and carbon dioxide is accomplished through the combined efforts of the
   a. respiratory, neurological, and cardiovascular systems
   b. respiratory, endocrine, and cardiovascular systems
   c. respiratory, endocrine, and neurological systems
   d. respiratory, neurological, and integumentary systems

623   2. A situation that causes parents to be most frightened would be seeing their child
   a. have an IV started
   b. have an X-ray done
   c. restrained
   d. in respiratory difficulty

623   3. An inflammatory condition of the lungs is called
   a. bronchitis   c. pleurisy
   b. cystic fibrosis   d. pneumonia

624   4. When treating a child with cystic fibrosis, the parents may exhibit extreme anxiety. The nurse may refer the parents to a
   a. respiratory therapist
   b. social worker
   c. genetic counselor
   d. dietitian

628   5. A life threatening condition that causes edema, which may obstruct the airway, is
   a. bronchitis   c. bronchiolitis
   b. epiglottitis   d. laryngitis

629　　6. The age at which a child is most at risk for foreign body aspiration is

　　　　　a.　4 months–12 years

　　　　　b.　6 months–6 years

　　　　　c.　4 months–4 years

　　　　　d.　6 months–4 years

631　　7. Mary, age 5, tells her mother she can't swallow. Mary also has a slight fever and some respiratory difficulty. The mother suspects Mary has

　　　　　a.　pharyngitis　　　　c.　strep throat

　　　　　b.　laryngitis　　　　　d.　epiglottitis

634　　8. One of the classic symptoms of asthma is

　　　　　a.　stridor

　　　　　b.　inspiratory wheezing

　　　　　c.　rales

　　　　　d.　expiratory wheezing

634　　9. To improve the respiratory status of a child with asthma, the nurse must be able to do all but

　　　　　a.　give oxygen as ordered

　　　　　b.　order the IV infusion

　　　　　c.　elevate the head of the bed

　　　　　d.　provide a calm and quiet environment

635　　10. The Mantoux test is done to check for

　　　　　a　cystic fibrosis　　　　c.　tuberculosis

　　　　　b.　pneumonia　　　　　d.　asthma

FILL IN THE BLANK

Complete the following statements.

624　　1. The sweat test done to diagnose cystic fibrosis checks for an increase in _Sodium_ and _Chloride_ levels.

626　　2. The term used to describe acute infectious diseases such as laryngitis or tracheitis is known as _Croup_ . _LTB_

630　　3. The term used to describe a nosebleed is _epistaxis_

630　　4. Nasopharyngitis is also known as a _common cold_ .

5. Fluid intake in children with respiratory disease can be encouraged by offering noncitrus fruit drinks, _____ and _____ .

MATCHING
Match the terms in the left column with their definitions in the right column.

634	9	a. nasal shiner	1.	increased respiratory rate
623	6	b. retractions	2.	fatty stools
631	5	c. snoring	3.	high pitched sound created by a narrowing of the airway
634	10	d. rhinitis	4.	stimulus
623	8	e. dyspnea	5.	adenoiditis
624	2	f. steatorrhea	6.	visible drawing in of the skin of the neck and chest
627	3	g. stridor	7.	wiping the nose with the back of the hand
634	7	h. nasal salute	8.	respiratory difficulty
634	4	i. trigger	9.	swollen eyes
623	1	j. tachypnea	10.	inflammation of the mucous membrane

EXERCISE

Give the rationale for the following treatment protocols for providing care to patients with respiratory diseases.

Treatment	Rationale
Oxygen	
Fluid therapy	
Airway support	
Rest	
Bronchodilators	~~epinephrine~~ (Adrenalin)
Antibiotics	pencillian erythromycin
Humidification	
Expectorants	Robitussin

CHAPTER 39

Digestive and Metabolic Conditions

MULTIPLE CHOICE
Select the one best answer.

638   1. The digestive system enables the body to
   a.   transport nutrients
   b.   circulate nutrients
   c.   metabolize nutrients
   d.   manufacture vitamin D

640   2. Since there may be a chance a baby could develop thrush, the nurse should instruct the mother to report the color of the baby's tongue if it has
   a.   cheesy, white patches
   b.   red patches only
   c.   moist, pink patches
   d.   white and red patches

640   3. Normal newborns by the age of 6 weeks cry about
   a.   2 hours per day
   b.   1 hour per day
   c.   4 hours per day
   d.   3 hours per day

641   4. Winter outbreaks of diarrhea in children in hospitals and day-care centers are caused by all of the following viruses except
   a.   herpes virus   c.   enterovirus
   b.   Norwalk virus   d.   rotavirus

645   5. The most frequent cause of intestinal obstruction during the first two years of life is
- a. Hirschsprung's disease
- b. paralytic ileus
- c. intussusception
- d. pyloric stenosis

650   6. A limited production of insulin by the pancreas causes insulin-dependent diabetes (IDDM), which results in
- a. loss of glucose to the cells and hyperglycemia
- b. increase of glucose in cells and hypoglycemia
- c. loss of fat to the cells and hyperglycemia
- d. increase of fat in the cells and hypoglycemia

650   7. Excessive thirst is known as
- a. polyuria
- b. glycosuria
- c. polydipsia
- d. polyphagia

651   8. Important factors that must be included in teaching a family about diabetes include all but how to
- a. monitor diet
- b. recognize hypoglycemia
- c. measure blood glucose levels
- d. measure urine glucose levels

649   9. If appendicitis is untreated, the appendix may rupture causing
- a. stomatitis
- b. gastritis
- c. gastroenteritis
- d. peritonitis

648   10. Foreign body ingestion is most common in
- a. infants
- b. toddlers
- c. school-age children
- d. adolescents

FILL IN THE BLANK
Complete the following statements.

640   1. A common disease of the oral cavity in infants is _____ , which creates a thick, cheesy, _____ coating on the tongue.

640   2. The typical position for colicky babies is to _____ their legs _____ to their chests.

642   3. The clinical sign of dehydration in an infant under 12 months of age is
Sunken fontanells & eyes

642   4. Dehydration can result from ___fever___, ___sweating___, and diarrhea.

645   5. When a newborn fails to pass meconium, the condition may be
Hirschsprung

645   6. In cases of intussusception the bowel movement may be normal followed two to three days later by a stool described as ___current jelly___ stool.

646   7. Most ___umbilical___ hernias close spontaneously by the time the child is ___2___ to ___3___ years of age.

651   8. The chemical breakdown of fats in metabolism leads to the buildup of ___Ketone___ bodies.

648   9. The treatment of children with high lead levels in the blood is called ___Chelation___ therapy. An agent is administered that binds with ___lead___ to prevent its ___absorption___ by the body.

649-650   10. A parent or nurse may suspect intussusception has occurred when a child suddenly develops ___severe___ abdominal pain accompanied by abdominal distention and ___bstned dk blood, current jelly___ stool.

MATCHING
Match the term in the left column with the definition in the right column.

640   _10_   a. thrush   1. increase in the frequency and water of the stool

640   _6_   b. colic   2. recurrent regurgitation or vomiting

640–641   _1_   c. diarrhea   3. excessive loss of body fluid

645   _7_   d. Hirschsprung's disease   4. narrowing of the stomach sphincter

642   _3_   e. dehydration   5. helminths

643   _2_   f. GER (gastroesophageal reflux)   6. unexplained crying

643   _4_   g. pyloric stenosis   7. hypertonic bowel

646   _5_   h. intestinal parasites   8. mental retardation

649   _9_   i. appendicitis   9. most common cause of surgery in children

648   _8_   j. lead poisoning   10. infection of the oral cavity

ACTIVITIES

640   1. Outline a plan of care for parents who have a colicky baby. Include how you would
        describe how a baby would position themselves, possible causes and techniques to
        quiet the infant.

648   2. List six sources of lead poisoning.

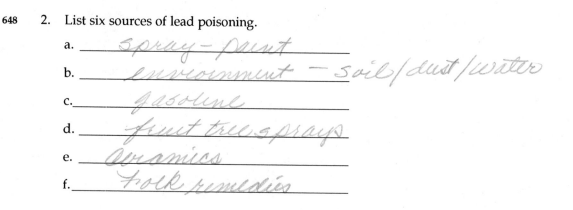

a. _____ Spray-paint _____

b. _____ environment — soil/dust/water

c. _____ gasoline _____

d. _____ fruit tree sprays _____

e. _____ Ceramics _____

f. _____ folk remedies _____

3. Marietta, age 10, is brought to the doctor's office by her mother, Mrs. C.

Mrs C reports that her daughter is losing weight and that Marietta had a respiratory infection about two weeks ago. In addition, she states that Marietta is urinating frequently and drinking unusual amounts of water. The doctor does a blood test and schedules Marietta for a glucose tolerance test. He tells the mother he suspects she may have diabetes mellitus.

The doctor wants you to schedule a family meeting to explain diabetes mellitus, the diagnostic testing, the symptoms, treatment, and diet. The educational program needs to consider that this is a 10-year-old child.

CHAPTER

40

Genitourinary Conditions

MULTIPLE CHOICE
Select the one best answer.

660   1. A congenital anomaly of male infants in which the urethral meatus is located on the ventral surface of the penis is known as

    a. hydrocele   c. epispadias

    b. hypospadias   d. cryptorchidism

660   2. A good diversionary activity for a 3-year-old postoperative child would be to

    a. do 500-piece puzzle

    b. listen to popular music

    c. play video games

    d. watch television

660   3. When one or both testicles fail to descend into the scrotal sac, the condition is known as

    a. hydrocele   c. epispadias

    b. hypospadias   d. cryptorchidism

661   4. The most common genitourinary disorder in childhood is

    a. cryptorchidism   c. cystitis

    b. urinary tract infection   d. glomerulonephritis

664   5. Excessive amounts of protein are produced and excreted in the urine in the condition known as

    a. Wilm's tumor

    b. glomerulonephritis

    c. nephrotic syndrome

    d. renal failure

666   6. Susan, age 10, is brought to the doctor's office with symptoms such as oliguria, dehydration, edema, and hypertension. After taking a history, the doctor orders tests to rule out
       a. cystitis
       b. glomerulonephritis
       c. renal failure
       d. urinary tract infection

665   7. A condition that may occur 10–14 days after a strep throat is
       a. urinary tract infection
       b. glomerulonephritis
       c. renal failure
       d. cystitis

670   8. The incubation period for gonorrhea is
       a. unknown   c. 3 to 5 days
       b. 3 weeks   d. 1 week

670   9. The most common cause of nongonococcal urethritis is
       a. *Chlamydia trachomatis*
       b. herpes simplex
       c. *Streptococcus*
       d. *Treponema pallidum*

671   10. Acylovir is the drug of choice to treat
       a. syphilis   c. herpes simplex
       b. gonorrhea   d. chlamydia

FILL IN THE BLANK
Complete the following statements.

660   1. A hydrocele is a condition in which _fluid_ from the _peritoneal_ cavity surrounds the testicle.

660   2. One of the complications that may occur in untreated cryptorchidism is _infertility_ .

661 3. The nurse should teach parents that children who have urinary tract infections should avoid __*tight nylon*__ underwear and __*synthetic*__ materials close to the body.

664 4. The cardinal sign of nephrotic syndrome is __*edema*__, which occurs because of __*poor renal perfusion*__ *age 2-3*

666 5. In renal failure, it is most important for the nurse to monitor __*I&O*__ and __*electrolytes*__

665 6. The diet of choice in glomerulonephritis is ___*↓*___ sodium and ___*↓*___ protein.

668 7. Adolescents are especially at risk for __*STD*__.

668 8. One of the causes of STD may be __*fail*__ to use protection.

MATCHING
Match the terms in the left column with their definitions in the right column.

667 __8__ a. enuresis 1. abnormal backflow of urine to the ureters

666 __3__ b. oliguria 2. decrease in the amount of protein in the blood

664 __7__ c. hypoalbuminemia 3. decrease in urinary output

666 __10__ d. hypovolemia 4. blood in the urine

661 __1__ e. vesicouretal reflux 5. painful urination

664 __9__ f. hyperlipidemia 6. protein in the urine

661 __5__ g. dysuria 7. abnormal low levels of albumin in blood

664 __4__ h. hematuria 8. involuntary urination

664 __2__ i. hypoproteinemia 9. abnormally high levels of lipids in plasma

664 __6__ j. proteinuria 10. diminished blood flow

SHORT ANSWER

661   1. List three conditions that may predispose a child to a urinary tract infection.

     a. *Urinary stasis*

     b. *obstruction*

     c. *Vesicoureteral*

661   2. List six strategies to teach parents to prevent urinary tract infections.

     a. *Clothes - cotton*

     b. *hygiene*

     c. *bath - no bubble*

     d. *↑ fluids*

     e. *wipe F to b*

     f. *(void after intercourse)*
     empty bladder frequently

667   3. List five guidelines for parents of children with enuresis.

     a. *Restrict fluids after supper*

     b. *alarm*

     c. *freq visit to bathroom bed*

     d. *Bladder stretching exercises*

     e. *Rewards*

ACTIVITY

668–671 You are asked to speak to a local ninth-grade high school class regarding sexually transmitted diseases. Outline an educational program to include four major sexually transmitted diseases. Include causes, symptoms, treatments, complications of the disease, prevention, and the public health risk.

Musculoskeletal Conditions

MULTIPLE CHOICE

Select the one best answer.

676 1. Danny Ryan, age 8 months, has acetabular dysplasia. You explain to his parents that this means
   a. acetabulum is shallow; femoral head is dislocated
   b. acetabulum is shallow; femoral head is in place
   c. head of femur is partially displaced
   d. head of femur is dislocated from acetabulum

676 2. Indicators of hip dysplasia include
   a. even gluteal folds, uneven knee height
   b. even gluteal folds, even knee height
   c. uneven gluteal folds, uneven knee height
   d. uneven gluteal folds, even knee height

676 3. A congenital deformity in which the foot is twisted out of its normal position is known as
   a. torticollis   c. rickets
   b. dysplasia   d. talipes

677 4. Muscular dystrophy symptoms include
   a. difficulty in running, hip displacement, pseudohypertrophy
   b. hip placement, difficulty in bicycle riding, pseudohypertrophy
   c. hip displacement, difficulty in running, frequent falls
   d. difficulty in running, frequent falls, pseudohypertrophy

678 5. A condition that may occur in school-age children that involves a loss of circulation to the femoral head is known as

  a. torticollis
  c. acetabular dysplasia
  b. Legg-Calvé Perthes disease
  d. juvenile rheumatoid arthritis

679 6. Michael, age 7, came home from school with a fever, irritability, and some pain in his ankle. Upon examination by the doctor, his ankle was warm to the touch. The doctor states he must rule out

  a. a viral infection
  c. osteomyelitis
  b. juvenile arthritis
  d. a sprained ankle

682 7. The most common site of childhood fracture treated in a hospital is the

  a. shoulder
  c. wrist
  b. humerus
  d. femur

684 8. Traction devices help to do all of the following except

  a. reduce dislocations
  b. reduce inflammation
  c. prevent contracture deformities
  d. provide rest for an extremity

686 9. When caring for the child in traction, the nurse should

  a. check pulse below affected area and compare with opposite extremity
  b. not check pulses to avoid an increase in pressure
  c. check pulse above affected area and compare with opposite extremity
  d. check pulse of affected area and compare with opposite extremity

687 10. Treatment for scoliosis may include use of a brace fitted from neck to

  a. knees worn continuously
  b. hips worn 2 hours on and 2 hours off
  c. knees worn 2 hours on and 2 hours off
  d. hips worn continuously

FILL IN THE BLANK

Complete the following statements.

675 1. A child's growth may be affected by injury to the _epyphyseal_

676 2. To abduct the hip in hip dysplasia in a 6-month-old, you may pin ___3___ or more cloth _diapers_ front to back.

677   3. To treat torticollis, you must use ___passive___ exercise to stretch the ___sternocleido-mastoid___ muscle.

677   4. Duchenne's muscular dystrophy usually occurs in ___boys___ between the age of ___3___ and ___5___ years old.

682   5. A break in a bone is called a ___fracture___.

682   6. A wet cast is handled by the ___palm___ portion of the hand to avoid ___indentation___ which may cause ___pressure___ on the skin.

686   7. In skeletal traction, the site where the wire or pin is inserted may be prone to ___infection___.

686   8. In caring for a patient in traction, it is critical that weights ___hang freely___.

688   9. Osteosarcoma is a ___rapid___ growing ___tumor___ of the bone.

688   10. The most common primary site of osteosarcoma is usually the ___distal femur___.

MATCHING
Match the terms in the left column with their definitions in the right column.

676   __3__   a. Ortolani's sign   1. increased curvature of the spine

677   __5__   b. pseudohypertrophy   2. self-climbing movement using arm muscles

677   __1__   c. lordosis   3. click heard as femur enters the acetabulum

685   __8__   d. Russell's traction   4. pulling of a ligament

677   __7__   e. rickets   5. muscle fibers replaced by fatty deposits

687   __10__   f. scoliosis   6. use of weights and pulleys to realign bone fragments

678   __2__   g. Gower's sign   7. bones weakened and bent out of shape

679   __4__   h. strain   8. skin traction

679   __9__   i. sprain   9. muscle injury caused by overstretching

684   __6__   j. traction   10. S-shaped curvature of the spine

LABELING

685–686 Name the traction illustrated in the following figures. Indicate whether it is a form of skin or skeletal traction, and provide a short description of its use.

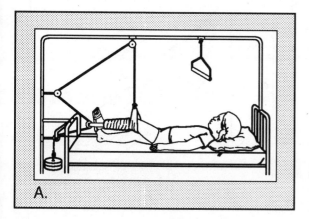

A.

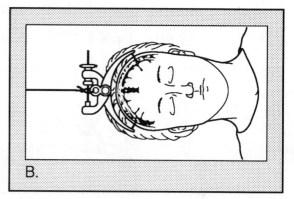

B.

Name:_____

Skin or Skeletal: _____

_____

_____

_____

_____

Name: _____

Skin or Skeletal: _____

_____

_____

_____

_____

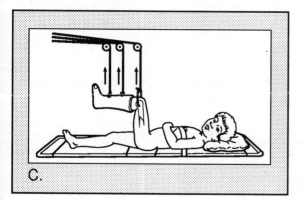

C.

Name:_____

Skin or Skeletal: _____

_____

_____

_____

_____

D.

Name: _____

Skin or Skeletal: _____

_____

_____

_____

_____

E.

F.

Name:_____   Name: _____

Skin or Skeletal: _____   Skin or Skeletal: _____

_____   _____

_____   _____

_____   _____

_____   _____

ACTIVITIES

679–681 1. Michael, age 8, is admitted to the hospital with osteomyelitis. He is upset because he was supposed to be in a soccer tournament. Develop a care plan for Michael that includes discharge planning.

Problem	Nursing Intervention
Anxiety and fear	

Problem	Nursing Intervention
Pain	
Lack of activity	
Risk of infection	
Prevention of recurrence	

684   2. Danny, age 6, broke his arm and had a cast applied. As the nurse in the emergency room, what instructions would give Danny? What instructions would give the parents?

CHAPTER

42

Neurological Conditions

MULTIPLE CHOICE
Select the one best answer.

693 1. The nervous system is responsible for all except
   a. conduction pathway
   b. motor function
   c. circulatory pathway
   d. conscious thought and memory

694 2. A neural tube defect in which there is a sac containing meninges, spinal fluid, and neural tissue is called
   a. meningocele
   b. myelomeningocele
   c. hydrocephalus
   d. spina bifida occulta

697 3. Children with loss of coordination in standing, walking, and who have a wide-based gait have
   a. dyskinetic cerebral palsy
   b. spastic cerebral palsy
   c. mixed-type cerebral palsy
   d. ataxic cerebral palsy

696 4. Patterns of disability that involve only one extremity are known as
   a. hemiplegia   c. quadreparesis
   b. monoplegia   d. paraplegia

236

700   5. Margaret, age 10, is brought to the doctor's office. Her mother explains that the teacher has sent home a note stating that Margaret appears to be daydreaming quite a lot. The doctor must rule out

    a. tonic-clonic seizure disorders

    b. absence seizure disorders

    c. myoclonic seizure disorders

    d. atonic seizure disorders

704   6. In the initial treatment of children with meningitis,

    a. fluids are increased to reduce intracranial pressure

    b. fluide are decreased to reduce intracranial pressure

    c. fluids are withheld to avoid vomiting

    d. 1,500 cc of fluid are given to reduce fever

712   7. The diagnostic test to determine Reye's syndrome is

    a. EEG

    b. CAT scan

    c. liver biopsy

    d. lumbar puncture

713   8. A pediatric brain tumor that may be cystic or benign is known as

    a. brain-stem glioma

    b. cerebellar astrocytoma

    c. ependymoma

    d. medulla blastoma

705   9. Since the head is larger in proportion to the rest of the body, children often fall from their beds during

    a. infancy   c. preschool age

    b. toddlerhood   d. school age

710   10. A hemorrhage that occurs between the dura mater and cerebrum is known as a(an)

    a. epidural hemorrhage

    b. subdural hemorrhage

    c. intracranial hemorrhage

    d. subarachnoid hemorrhage

FILL IN THE BLANK

Complete the following statements.

694   1. When the neural tube fails to close during fetal development, the condition is known as a neural tube defect or _____.

695–696   2. A nonprogressive neurological disorder that affects movement or posture and occurs in infancy is known as _____.

699   3. Treatment approaches for cerebral palsy include casts, _____ , and _____ devices.

698   4. An uncontrolled episode of excess electrical activity is known as a _____ .

698   5. Febrile seizures occur in children between the ages of _____ months and _____ years.

701   6. In infants under 18 months of age, the most significant sign of meningitis is a _____ fontanel.

706–707   7. When caring for a child with meningitis, it is important to remember movement of the _____ and _____ is most _____.

710   8. Inflammation of the brain is _____.

710–711   9. In Reye's syndrome, the _____ fails to convert _____ to urea, resulting in toxic _____ . There appears to be a possible link between the use of _____ and Reye's syndrome.

705   10. The most common malignant tumor in children is _____ , which may be located in the _____ cavity.

MATCHING

Match the term in the left column with the definition in the right column.

696   _____   a.   apraxia   1.   increased resistance to passive movement

697   _____   b.   athetosis movement   2.   flailing, circular movement

696   _____   c.   spastic cerebral palsy   3.   stiff neck

697   _____   d.   hemiballismus   4.   generalized tonic-clonic seizures; remains unconsciousness between seizures

700   _____   e.   myoclonic seizure   5.   unable to initiate voluntary movement

697   _____   f.   nuchal rigidity   6.   slow, rhythmic twisting or abnormal posture

697   _____   g.   dystonia   7.   extremely high muscle tone in any position

699   _____   h.   status epilepticus   8.   involuntary movements that look purposeful

700   _____   i.   automatisms   9.   slow, writhing, wormlike movements

697   _____   j.   rigidity   10.   brief jerks of a muscle or group of muscles

ACTIVITIES

696   1.   List three causes of cerebral palsy.

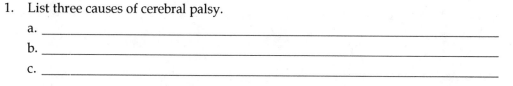

a. _____

b. _____

c. _____

698–703   2.   Eileen, age six, has been diagnosed with tonic-clonic seizure disorder. Eileen's parents ask you to explain what happens. She is in first grade and her parents want to know what to tell family and friends about Eileen's condition.

701, 704,   3. Write a protocol for treatment or nursing care plan for Vinny, age 16, who is
706–707   admitted to the adolescent unit with meningitis in October. Vinny is a star player on
               his school football team.

CHAPTER

43

Conditions of the Blood and Blood Forming Organs

MULTIPLE CHOICE
Select the one best answer.

719   1. The type of blood cells that become elevated in allergic conditions are known as

     a. neutrophils   c. lymphocytes

     b. eosinophils   d. monocytes

720   2. Carolyn, age 8, has iron deficiency anemia and is taking ferrous sulfate tablets. You must instruct her that her stools will be

     a. brown   c. yellow

     b. grey   d. black *or green*

722   3. A common occurrence in adolescents with sickle cell anemia is

     a. pallor and jaundice

     b. black, tarry stools

     c. leg ulcers

     d. pale conjunctiva

720   4. Situations that can result in hypoxia in patients with anemia include

     a. hot, humid weather and exercise

     b. airplane ride

     c. walking through fall leaves

     d. climbing up a mountain

722   5. Johnny, age 4, has fallen off his bicycle. His mother becomes very agitated. The elbow joint appears swollen. After a blood test, the doctor suspects hemophilia because
       a. the platelets are elevated
       b. activated partial thromboplastin is prolonged
       c. bleeding and clotting are shortened
       d. red blood cells are increased

724   6. Leukemia occurs when there is a rapid growth of immature white blood cells. Diagnosis is confirmed by
       a. white blood test
       b. partial thromboplastin time
       c. bone marrow aspiration
       d. complete blood count

724   7. The treatment for leukemia includes all but
       a. chemotherapeutic agents
       b. intrathecal methotrexate
       c. bone marrow transplant
       d. radiation

725   8. In idiopathic thrombocytopenia, there is a decrease in
       a. platelets   c. erythrocytes
       b. lymphocytes   d. neutrophils

730   9. Hodgkin's disease occurs most often in
       a. infants   c. toddlers
       b. school-age children d. adolescents

730   10. One of the major symptoms in Hodgkin's disease is
       a. swelling in joints
       b. lymphadenopathy
       c. cardiomegaly
       d. hepatomegaly

FILL IN THE BLANK
Complete the following statements.

720   1. Young children are prone to iron deficiency anemia due to their high intake of milk, which _____ the absorption of iron.

719   2. A normal red blood cell lasts _____ days; the life span of a sickle cell

               is_____ to _____ days.

721   3. Sickle cell crisis in children causes pain that may be controlled

               by_____ .

725   4. The drugs used to treat leukemia may cause _____

               and _____ .

725   5. In most cases, the cause of idiopathic thrombocytopenia purpura

               is_____ .

THE STORY OF THE GOOD FLUID

Write the missing word to complete the story.

Blood is formed by a combination of many things—
Plasma, WBC, RBC, and _____ .
Does it have a familiar ring?

Everyone has a job to do to keep things in order.
If they don't, you can develop a blood _____ .

The little cell that circulates carrying _____ to and fro
Is known as an _____ you know.

White blood cells are needed for _____ .
They are the body system's way to fight _____ .

When you are injured, you need platelets to help form a _____ .
Otherwise you would _____ quite a lot .

In the plasma protein, you have nutrients and electrolytes that keep the
acid-base _____ just _____ .

Be sure your blood gets its vitamins and _____ .
And it will keep the body in good _____ .

ACTIVITIES

721   1. Describe three types of sickle cell crises, along with their symptoms and required treatment.

723–729   2. Missy, age 10, has been diagnosed with leukemia. Her parents are blaming themselves because she had a cold a few weeks ago, and they didn't take her to the physician. Develop a nursing care plan for Missy.

Problem	Goal	Nursing Intervention
Anxiety of Missy caused by intrusive diagnostic tests		

Problem	Goal	Nursing Intervention
Anxiety of parents		
Immuno-suppression		

Emotional and Behavioral Conditions

MULTIPLE CHOICE

Select the one best answer.

737   1. Symptoms of children diagnosed with failure to thrive syndrome include

   a.   minimal eye contact, apathy, and stranger anxiety

   b.   eye contact, alertness, lack of stranger anxiety

   c.   minimal eye contact, apathy, lack of stranger anxiety

   d.   minimal eye contact, hypoalertness, stranger anxiety

737   2. Frank and Mary C are seen with their infant daughter Fran. You know bonding is occurring because of all the following except

   a.   there is no direct eye contact

   b.   they are touching the infant

   c.   they are examining the infant's toes

   d.   they are talking to the baby

739   3. You may suspect that Danny, age 6, has attention deficit disorder because his teacher report she

   a.   finishes his work, but is slow

   b.   fidgets and squirms in his seat

   c.   acts as class monitor, opening and closing the door

   d.   he asks questions frequently

744   4. Another form of separation anxiety in a child may be exhibited as

   a.   attention deficit disorder

   b.   failure to thrive syndrome

   c.   an eating disorder

   d.   school phobia

745   5. Wayne is 13 years old, 5 feet 8 inches tall, and weighs 240 pounds. The doctor states he is obese because his weight is_____ above ideal for his height.

     a.   5%–10%

     b.   10%–20%

     c.   20%–30%

     d.   30%–40%

746   6. Symptoms of anorexia nervosa include all but

     a.   bruising

     b.   lanugo

     c.   dry skin

     d.   normal menstrual cycle

747   7. The adolescent with bulimia usually maintains

     a.   weight 20% over normal

     b.   normal weight

     c.   weight 20% below normal

     d.   weight 10% below normal

748   8. In a discussion with 16-year-old Nicole, Nicole makes the following statement that may indicate depression:

     a.   "I'm much too fat, and my hair is terrible."

     b.   "I don't want to do anything in life. Everything rots."

     c.   "I don't have a boyfriend for the junior prom. What am I going to do?"

     d.   "My hair looks terrible, and I have nothing to wear. I'm not going out."

750   9. You may suspect a child has a "crack habit" if he develops symptoms of

     a.   impaired ability to concentrate

     b.   flashbacks and personality changes

     c.   chronic sinus and upper respiratory congestion

     d.   gastritis and peptic ulcer disease

749–750   10. Which group would be most effective in educating Johnny, age 14, about the devastating effects of substance abuse?

     a.   M.A.D.D.   c.   S.A.D.D.

     b.   D.A.R.E.   d.   A. A.

FILL IN THE BLANK

Complete the following statements.

737   1. When baby Margaret was born, her weight was 9 pounds. Today at the pediatric clinic, her weight is 14 pounds. She is 12 months old. A possible diagnosis is _____ syndrome.

737   2. In order for children to achieve self-esteem, they must learn to _____ . When bonding and attachment do not occur between parents and child, the child may view the world as _____ and _____ .

744   3. A parent may suspect a child has school phobia because during the week the child frequently has a stomach ache, which is _____ on Sundays.

745   4. A child may be overweight yet be _____ because the food she eats lacks _____ value.

746   5. Maureen, age 12, is hardly eating anything because of fear of being _____. She may develop _____ .

747   6. A teenager who has bulimia nervosa exhibits _____ and _____ .

748   7. Teenagers who are diagnosed with depression exhibit signs of anguish or _____ and lack of interest or _____ .

748   8. Suicide has become the _____ leading cause of death in young adults ages 15–24.

749   9. In the treatment plan of an adolescent who is at risk of committing suicide, the adolescent should be asked _____ whether he of she is considering _____ and if they have a plan.

750   10. In dealing with the adolescent with a substance abuse problem, the nurse must be _____ and _____ .

SHORT ANSWER

736   1. List five general principles that will assist the nurse in caring for a child with an emotional disorder.

a. _____

b. _____

c. _____

d. _____

e. _____

739   2. Describe five guidelines to include in a treatment plan for Danny, age 6, who has attention deficit disorder.

a. _____

b. _____

c. _____

d. _____

e. _____

749-750   3. List support groups for adolescents with a substance abuse problem.